T0212403

Havana Syndrome

Robert W. Baloh · Robert E. Bartholomew

Havana Syndrome

Mass Psychogenic Illness and the Real Story Behind the Embassy Mystery and Hysteria

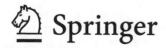

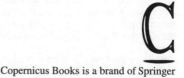

Copernicus Books is a brand of Springer

Robert W. Baloh
Department of Neurology and
Head and Neck Surgery
David Geffen School of Medicine at UCLA
Los Angeles, CA
USA

Robert E. Bartholomew
Psychological Medicine
University of Auckland
Auckland
New Zealand

ISBN 978-3-030-40745-2   ISBN 978-3-030-40746-9   (eBook)
https://doi.org/10.1007/978-3-030-40746-9

This Copernicus imprint is published by the registered company Springer Nature Switzerland AG
The registered company address is: Gewerbestrasse 11, 6330 Cham, Switzerland

Foreword I

The so-called acoustic attack on diplomats in the American Embassy in Havana, Cuba, beginning in late 2016, caught the attention of the world media. Those affected mostly reported hearing an unusual sound, often accompanied by pressure or vibration. Sometimes, the noise caused cognitive symptoms such as memory problems. The American Government blamed an acoustic weapon, although sound experts cast doubt on this as a likely cause. A report in the respected *Journal of the American Medical Association* evaluating the staff affected seemed initially to add further support for physical damage from some kind of external source.

Enter Robert Bartholomew and Robert Baloh. Dr. Bartholomew is the world's leading international expert on mass psychogenic illness. He has been an active researcher in the field for the past 25 years and conducted a meticulous analysis of the Havana episode, drawing on all the available material and his considerable experience of similar illness outbreaks. Dr. Baloh has conducted a similar analysis as a pioneer in neurotology – the study of neurological disorders of the ear. A distinguished professor of Neurology and Head and Neck Surgery at the David Geffen School of Medicine, UCLA, he has served as director of the UCLA Neurotology Testing Laboratory since 1974 and devised tests that are used by neurologists around the world.

This book is the result of their investigation and detective work. It is a cogent and convincing analysis that mass psychogenic illness is the likely cause of the Havana incident. Mass psychogenic illnesses are fascinating phenomena and are much more common than most people realize. Typically, they occur in closed social groups, like schools, army barracks, or factories. Often, there is a backdrop of raised levels of stress and anxiety. These illnesses are set off by unusual environmental agents like a smell or insect. The Havana episode is an enthralling case, as it brings together the political background of what was occurring in Cuban-American relations at the time with the search for a cause of unusual symptoms that also spread to other embassies. This book represents the author's dogged determination and focus to get to the bottom of what happened in Havana. It is a lively and enthralling read. The world needs more Bartholomews and Balohs who question and test official explanations and are prepared to roll their sleeves up and dig into these fascinating cases. The results of their analysis not only shed light on this case but provide a greater understanding of human behavior.

Keith J. Petrie
Professor of Health Psychology
Auckland University School of Medicine
Auckland, New Zealand

Foreword II

In a concise and engagingly-written volume, Doctors Baloh and Bartholomew make the case that the so-called "Havana syndrome" is simply the latest entry in a long and storied history of severe illness whose origin is psychological (psychogenic) rather than physical. Such illnesses, though extremely common, are understood very poorly by both the medical profession and the public. Rather than being treated with empathy and compassion, the sufferers and victims often are stigmatized.

The striking and impressive finding from the carefully-researched manuscript is that poor information – and in some cases deliberately false or misleading information – leads to real physical suffering and, in the case of the Havana illnesses, to global political consequences. While these authors wisely stay away from considering political motives, it is also clear that the individual agendas of policy makers have made important contributions to the problem, as powerful players such as the US Department of State release broad public announcement based almost strictly on speculation.

The events in Havana, and the domino consequences that followed, were propagated by well-meaning physicians, by shady characters pursuing narrow fiscal interests, by journalists who are eager for a story (but short on thoughtful investigation), and by a generally credulous and uncritical public that chooses to trust its media and its government. What we learn from this book is that this is the very climate in which to brew a perfect storm of hysteria.

Baloh and Bartholomew go far beyond Havana to make their case. They chart psychogenic mass illnesses through centuries of experience. They show both that history is chock full of examples of disorders having essentially all of the features of the Havana syndrome and, disturbingly, that even today our impulse is to discount these historical lessons and instead to concoct fanciful explanations such as weaponized sounds, if only to avoid labeling the victims of these syndromes as hysterics. In so doing, we not only amplify the illnesses, but we fail the victims by excluding them from the insight treatments that might be effective.

This is an important book for professionals in journalism, for people in policy positions, for a lay audience seeking to gain insight into the reality of life in a mass media age, and for medical professionals who, once again, need to learn these lessons to care for their patients.

Mark S. Cohen
Professor of Psychiatry, Neurology, Radiology
Bioengineering, Psychology and Biomedical Physics
University of California Los Angeles
Los Angeles, CA, USA

Imagination frames events unknown, in wild, fantastic shapes of hideous ruin, and what it fears, creates.

–Hannah More (Hannah More, *The Poetical Works of Hannah More with an Account of Her Life*. London: Scott, Webster, and Geary; 1838: p. 73)

Contents

About the Authors

Robert W. Baloh is well known in the field of neurology. He is a distinguished professor of Neurology and Head and Neck Surgery at the David Geffen School of Medicine, UCLA. He has served as director of the Neurotology Testing Laboratory at the Ronald Reagan UCLA Medical Center since 1974. Author of 11 books and over 300 articles in peer-reviewed science journals, he is a pioneer in the study of the vestibular system: the part of the inner ear which helps people to maintain their sense of balance and spatial awareness. He has developed tests of vestibular function that are used by inner ear specialists around the world. His book *Clinical Neurophysiology of the Vestibular System*, written with Dr. Vicente Honrubia, is currently in its fourth edition and is the standard in the field. His other books include *Dizziness, Hearing Loss, and Tinnitus: The Essentials of Neurotology* (1984), *Neurotology* (1994), *Dizziness: Why Do You Feel Dizzy and What Will Help You Feel Better* (with Gregory T. Whitman), *Vertigo: Five Physician Scientists and the Quest for a Cure* (2017), and *Sciatica and Chronic Pain: Past, Present and Future* (2019).

Robert E. Bartholomew is a medical sociologist who has written extensively on the inappropriate placement of disease or disorder labels onto unpopular or unfamiliar behaviors. He has published on such topics as hoaxes, popular delusions, psychological disorders, the history of tabloid journalism, and pseudoscience and coined the term "exotic deviance" in the field of sociology. He began his career as a journalist for several New York State radio stations and has lived with the Malay people in Malaysia and Aborigines in the Tanami Desert of Central Australia. He completed his Ph.D. in Sociology from James Cook University in Australia and his Master's in Sociology from the State University of New York at Albany. He has published in over 60 peer-reviewed journals. Robert has been featured in a National Geographic series on modern myths and has appeared on The History Channel and Discovery Channel. A Fellow with the Center for Inquiry in Amherst, New York, he teaches History at Botany College in Auckland, New Zealand. His books include *American Intolerance: Our Dark History of Demonizing Immigrants* (with Anja Reumschüssel, 2018), *A Colorful History of Popular Delusions* (with Peter Hassall, 2015), and *Outbreak! The Encyclopedia of Extraordinary Social Behavior* (with Hilary Evans, 2009).

Mark S. Cohen did his undergraduate work at MIT and Stanford, and received his Ph.D. from the Rockefeller University. He worked on magnetic resonance imaging instrumentation at Siemens Medical and at Advanced NMR Systems then accepted a faculty position at Harvard/Massachusetts General Hospital, before moving to the University of California Los Angeles, where he is a professor of psychiatry, neurology, radiology, biomedical physics, psychology and bioengineering. Cohen performed pioneering studies that led to the invention of functional MRI and his work includes breakthroughs in digital signal processing, machine learning, electroencephalography, ultrasound and MRI.

Keith J. Petrie is the Head of Health Psychology at the University of Auckland in New Zealand. Of particular relevance to "Havana syndrome" is his research on the nocebo and placebo effect and how health worries about modern life and new technologies impact on well-being. He has participated in several studies examining the purported health effects of infrasound from wind turbines. An array of health complaints by people living in the vicinity of certain wind farms suggests that the expectation and framing of this new technology as hazardous is pivotal in generating a negative health response. Dr. Petrie is a Fellow of the Royal Society of New Zealand.

Chasing Ghosts in Cuba

If men define situations as real, they are real in their consequences.

–William Isaac Thomas [1]

It reads like the pages from a spy novel. State Department doctors uncover an attack on diplomats at the American Embassy in Havana, Cuba by a hostile foreign power using a mysterious new weapon that causes brain damage. Those affected are evacuated stateside for treatment. Their health problems are extensive: headaches, dizziness, nausea, and fatigue. Some describe being in a strange mental fog and have difficulty concentrating and remembering things. Many are confused and disoriented. Others have trouble walking, sleeping, and focusing their eyes. They complain of an array of ear problems: sensitivity to sound, tinnitus, pain, pressure, and hearing loss. Most concerning of all are the concussion-like symptoms. An eerie, high-pitched sound accompanies most of the attacks, described variously as piercing, buzzing, and grinding. One affected embassy diplomat told a journalist that it was "a very high-pitched sound" that resembled "a teapot on steroids" [2]. State Department representative Heather Nauert would later observe: "We have never seen this anyplace in the world before" [3]. There is concern that a new weapon has been developed and is being used against Americans, most likely by the Russians or Chinese with the knowledge of the government in Havana. The attacks spur the State Department to expel Cuban diplomats and threaten to shut down the Embassy. Reports also emerge of Canadian diplomats in Havana who are also affected by the mysterious attacks [4].

In early 2018, 15 months after the first reported attack, the case takes a new and dramatic twist as a team of neuroscientists at the University of Pennsylvania confirm the existence of concussion-like symptoms that damaged the American patients' brains from what they refer to as "an unknown energy source" [5]. The findings are published in the prestigious *Journal of the American Medical Association* and make headlines around the world. Who was behind these nefarious attacks? What was their purpose, and what was the strange new weapon? The *JAMA* study led to a flurry of sensational news stories confirming not only that the attacks had taken place but had

© Springer Nature Switzerland AG 2020
R. W. Baloh, R. E. Bartholomew, *Havana Syndrome*,
https://doi.org/10.1007/978-3-030-40746-9_1

caused brain trauma. It was no longer a question of 'if,' but 'who' was behind them. The *Los Angeles Times* proclaimed: "U.S. Diplomats Suffered Brain Injuries…" [6]. The *Washington Post* declared: "Neurological Injuries Found in U.S. Staff in Cuba" [7]. *Time* magazine carried the headline: "Cuba Denies Role in 'Sonic Attacks' that Left U.S. Diplomats with Brain Damage" [8]. The United Kingdom's second largest newspaper, the *Daily Mail*, reported: "Damning evidence Cuba's launched a sci-fi sonic weapon at America as…US diplomats are hit by hearing and memory loss – and even mild brain damage…" Its reporter, Tom Leonard, observed that he was hard-pressed to come up with "a more bizarre case of Cold War-style skullduggery since Bulgarian dissident Georgi Markov was assassinated in a London street with a poison-tipped umbrella in 1978" [9].

With publication of the study, it was clear that something sinister had happened. The State Department even emphasized that these were "medically confirmed symptoms" that had been verified by no less than eight doctors working at the University of Pennsylvania [10]. The media, the government and one of the world's most respected medical journals were all pointing in the same direction: US Embassy staff were the victims of a mysterious new weapon that had produced a never-before-seen syndrome. *There is only one problem with this story – it never happened.* There was no secret weapon, and there was no attack. At first glance, the claims appear to have merit, but dig deeper and look at the science behind these assertions, and it makes little sense. The claims are pseudoscience: a set of theories and claims that appear to be grounded in science and facts but do not follow the scientific method.

Havana 'Syndrome' Unmasked

In this book, we conclude that the mysterious 'new' illness that has baffled doctors and government officials, is part of a series of outbreaks dating back to ancient times: mass psychogenic illness. While there is no underlying disease, the symptoms are real and distressing. Imagine being told that you had just eaten rat poison. You might suddenly experience stomach pain, develop breathing problems and vomit, yet there is no underlying medical problem, only an idea. Psychogenic illness works in a similar way and is driven by suggestion and belief. You may be thinking: 'This is absurd! Mass psychogenic illness cannot cause concussion-like symptoms and brain abnormalities.' Not true. Victims commonly experience neurological complaints – abnormalities in brain function that often mimic *concussion-like symptoms*. This is very different from claiming there was brain damage. Reports that were leaked to the media prior to the publication of the 2018 *JAMA* study, claiming that many of the affected diplomats were suffering from mysterious white matter tract changes to their brains, turned out to be false. When the magnetic resonance imaging (MRI) results were released, a few had minor changes to their white matter tracts, but this would not be unusual for any group of normal subjects of that sample size. There is a big difference between claiming that there were brain *abnormalities* and asserting there was brain *damage*.

Mass psychogenic illness can be thought of as the placebo effect in reverse. It has long been known that people who are given a substance that has no therapeutic value such as a sugar pill, may feel better through the power of suggestion. The placebo effect will not lower cholesterol or heal diabetes, but it can change brain chemistry and physiology and how the patients react to their symptoms. It seems to work best on pain and stress-related conditions. More recently scientists have identified the nocebo effect, whereby subjects can make themselves sick solely through the power of belief. For instance, if a patient has negative expectations toward a treatment, it can elicit symptoms that reflect the anticipated outcome. Mass psychogenic illness is a functional disorder as it involves a disturbance of the normal functioning of the nervous system in response to stress. Outbreaks typically reflect the exposure scenario. Persons who believe they have been exposed to tainted food commonly experience abdominal pain, diarrhea, nausea, and vomiting, while those who think they have come into contact with toxic gas typically exhibit dizziness, itchy eyes, and breathing problems.

A second factor at work is reframing. Given the power of doctors to shape the presentation of symptoms through suggestion, many complaints that are common in the general population such as fatigue, dizziness, headaches, and memory problems, can become reframed to reflect what doctors and government authorities are telling them. Suddenly, someone who has been experiencing ambiguous aches and pains for years begins attributing their symptoms to some new illness category such as a sonic or microwave attack. These ongoing complaints are common: most general practitioners and neurologists would see them every day in their practices. Like mass psychogenic illness, they too are a form of functional disorder, but more individual than collective, caused by a malfunctioning or overstimulation of the nervous system. This condition is often prompted by stress. With the passage of time, these conditions tend to resolve on their own. British neurologist Jon Stone refers to both individual and collective forms of functional disorders as software problems [11].

As for the claim that 'Havana Syndrome' is unprecedented, it too is false. Many psychogenic outbreaks have involved victims who attributed their symptoms to sound waves. One famous example is 'acoustical shock' from the early days of the telephone, which was thought by some physicians to have induced *concussion-like symptoms*. Once people became used to talking on the telephone and grew accustomed to this strange new device, the condition gradually disappeared because concerns over its impact on health were a product of fear and human imagination. In fact, *concussion-like symptoms* have been reported in American soldiers returning home from every major conflict since modern doctors began keeping tabs on troops, from World War I to the fighting in Iraq and Afghanistan. Many were nowhere near exploding artillery shells. There is a growing consensus in the medical community that these symptoms were stress-related and psychogenic in nature. Yet, the lion's share of media coverage on 'Havana Syndrome' has focused on sensational claims about brain damage. Many openly ridicule the notion that mass psychogenic illness could be to blame. Not only is it the only plausible explanation, the illness clusters among embassy diplomats exhibit the telltale signs. As investigative journalist Jack Hitt observes: If you view the events in Havana as an attack, you need to look for something that is capable of producing the reported symptoms. "It would have to emit a sound that varied widely from listener to listener. It would have to strike only people who worked at the embassy. It would have to assail them wherever they happened to be, whether in their homes or staying at a hotel. It would have to produce a wide range of symptoms that seemed to bear no relation to one another." This led Hitt to the only conclusion that fit the facts: mass suggestion [12].

There are many misconceptions surrounding mass psychogenic illness. For instance, it is sometimes asserted that those affected have weak mental constitutions or are psychologically disturbed. Psychogenic illness can affect anyone. Most victims are normal, healthy people. It is a collective stress response that is not just 'all in their heads.' Those affected experience physical changes in the way their brains work. This is what fooled some of the early investigators looking at the American Embassy patients. They were seeing abnormalities in brain function that were confused with brain damage. Neurologists have found that patients suffering from common conditions like depression and chronic pain have discernible changes in their brains. Our beliefs and experiences can and do affect our brains by altering the connections and the way the brain transmits information as it reorganizes itself to adapt to new situations. MRIs of the brains of people with chronic depression have altered nerve pathways that connect different parts of the nervous system. But the brain is not static and over time can revert back to a more normal state of functioning. This is why the placebo effect is so powerful: if you believe you are getting better, it can trigger changes in your brain that may promote healing. However, if the patients from the Embassy in Cuba buy into claims that they have brain damage, it is likely to delay their recovery. It is also important to realize that while the media has dubbed the illness outbreak in Cuba 'Havana Syndrome,' it is clearly not. A syndrome is a group of symptoms that regularly occur together. In the Embassy patients, there is a significant variation in complaints from person to person. It is more accurately described as an illness. To avoid confusion, we have retained the term 'Havana Syndrome,' but placed it in quotation marks as it is a social construct.

This is the story of how much of the world came to believe in something that never happened. It is an extraordinary tale of international intrigue, flawed science, political ineptitude, and the mating habits of two most unlikely suspects: crickets and cicadas. While parts of the story border on the comical and at times are absurd, this saga has had far-reaching diplomatic repercussions as the fear and mistrust it has sown has threatened to undermine the future of Cuban-American relations. It has also undercut the institution of science itself as the ongoing public dispute among scientists over the cause of 'Havana Syndrome' has fostered confusion and skepticism. This book will not only help the diplomats in Cuba to better understand what happened to them, it can assist millions of others around the world who suffer from different forms of this condition. Learning about it and accepting the diagnosis is the key to recovery. Just as a set of beliefs caused their symptoms, reversing those beliefs can promote healing. It is imperative that the victims in Havana understand that any critical questioning of the official narrative is not intended to undermine their personal stories and credibility. Their symptoms and suffering are real, but they are not from a mysterious energy force, they are due to physiological changes in the brain that are triggered by chronic stress. The problem is, if a person accepts that they have a brain injury, it can hinder their recovery through the power of negative expectation. Conversely, if they come to accept that they are experiencing a collective stress response, it can act as a placebo and accelerate their recovery. Unfortunately, the literature on psychogenic outbreaks shows that when politics are involved, and the sufferers become political footballs, the prognosis for patients is poor. There is often a similar outcome when the media enter the fray. This is exactly what happened. For instance, Embassy personnel in Cuba were given strict instructions not to talk to the media. However, that rule was broken when it fit the State Department agenda. Some employees were given permission to talk about their symptoms to *The New Yorker* and other media outlets for one reason only: it supported the government's narrative that an attack took place. Incidentally, when *The New Yorker* article appeared, their reporter bought the government narrative, hook, line, and sinker, discussing the 'attacks' as if they had happened [13].

Mass psychogenic illness, also called mass hysteria, is one of the most fascinating and misunderstood conditions in all of medicine. Many physicians prefer the former term because of the negative connotations associated with "hysteria," which was initially thought to result from a "wandering uterus" and to only affect women. Both terms are used throughout the book for historical continuity, as only in recent times has mass psychogenic illness been preferred. We do so with the understanding that it refers to a psychophysiological (mind-body) illness that is equivalent to 'conversion disorder' and 'somatic symptom disorder,' affecting both men and women.

Mass hysteria involves the rapid spread of illness symptoms within a cohesive group, and has no organic basis. We will show that every key feature of the Havana illness has direct parallels with psychogenic illness, even down to the role of insects in triggering cases. Bugs have even been instrumental in the propagation of several episodes. There are hundreds of examples involving phantom assailants. There have been several recent cases where assailants were believed to have been agents acting on behalf of a hostile foreign power – again mirroring the events in Cuba. In short, the 'sonic attack' saga contains all of the elements of social contagion. New technologies have been fertile ground for the changing form of psychogenic outbreaks as episodes are driven by anxieties and prevailing fears. Soon after the invention of the radio, many people believed that the invisible waves were making them sick. When computer terminals became widespread by the early 1980s, some people were convinced that they were causing birth defects and miscarriages. More recently, fears that mobile phones and Wi-Fi would cause a spike in the number of brain tumors, have not materialized.

The Curious Case of Chris Allen

In April 2014, Chris Allen, a 33-year-old businessman from South Carolina, traveled to Havana for a weekend of sightseeing [14]. This was before travel restrictions were lifted by the Obama administration, so he booked the flight through Mexico using a Canadian travel company that recommended he stay at the Hotel Capri. A well-known hangout for mobsters before Cuba's 1959 revolution, the Capri was completely refurbished and reopened a few months earlier under joint ownership of Cuba's state-run tourism company and a Spanish hotel chain. After spending his first day sightseeing throughout the city, he checked into room 1414. Minutes after getting into bed Chris noticed numbness and tingling in his toes, and a pins and needles feeling similar to what happens if your arm goes to sleep after lying on it. The sensations gradually moved to his ankles and calves and into the fingertips. When he got out of bed, the tingling went away but soon returned, extending upward to his hands, arms and even his cheeks, ears, and neck. He eventually got to sleep, and the next day the tingling was gone, but that night when he got into bed, the numbness and tingling returned, stronger than ever. This time it did not go away, and the next morning he rushed to the airport and took the next available flight home. Arriving in South Carolina, he saw a series of neurologists. None could explain what happened. After extensive testing, doctors considered a range of possibilities from infections to toxins like ciguatoxin, a substance some Caribbean fish use to paralyze prey. All were ruled out. After 6 months, his symptoms gradually went away. "When you have these vague symptoms, sometimes all you can do is prove what it's not," said Allen's longtime physician, Dr. George Durst, "No one's smart enough to figure out what it was" [14]. Durst went on to note that he didn't think that Allen was imagining his symptoms and that they were probably coming from the central nervous system.

In September 2017, Allen began receiving phone calls from family and friends asking if he had seen the Associated Press report that the Hotel Capri was the site of several bizarre episodes of what US officials called "sonic attacks" causing neurological symptoms in Embassy staff? He wondered whether he had been a victim of such an attack even though he didn't recall hearing any sound at the time. Upon hearing the news of the Capri, he said: "I wanted to wave a flag and be like, I know this, I know what it is like to stay there and have something weird happen to your body and not be able to explain it" [14]. Allen contacted the Associated Press to see how he might get in touch with government officials about his experience but was told that the government was not interested in talking to potentially affected tourists. The AP journalist agreed with Allen that he might have been the first victim of the Cuban attacks since he was one of the first Americans to stay at the newly renovated building. They pointed out that the "clean-cut" young man who had worked with different Republican politicians could have looked like a spy to an outsider. The State Department did publish a warning that "assaults" had occurred in popular tourist hotels in Cuba including the Capri and that the US Government was no longer in a position to guarantee its citizens safety. They subsequently received reports from several American citizens who had visited Cuba and reported developing similar symptoms to those of the Embassy employees and their families, but they were directed to "consult a medical professional." The AP reported that since they began their coverage of the Cuban "attacks," they had been contacted by about three dozen American citizens who had visited Cuba and thought they had experienced the same phenomena encountered by the Embassy staff.

The Press Briefing

In July 2017, Steve Dorsey, a correspondent for CBS Radio News based in Washington DC, received a tip that something strange was happening to Americans working in Cuba. Employees at the US Embassy in Havana were becoming sick or injured under mysterious circumstances. Over the next few weeks, he pressed his sources for more detail [15]. Then on Wednesday afternoon, August 9, he walked into a State Department Press briefing, determined to find out more. "Can you tell us about the incidents that have been going on in Havana, affecting US Government workers there?" he asked. Heather Nauert confirmed the claims and admitted that for the past several months the Department had been accumulating evidence that staff working at the Embassy had been involved in "incidents" that "caused a variety of physical symptoms." She said that "some of our people have had the option of leaving Cuba as a result for medical reasons," and had done so. She refused to elaborate but said that because of these developments, on May 23 the State Department had expelled two diplomats from the Cuban Embassy in Washington [16]. Clearly, by virtue of these actions, this was a major diplomatic episode that was being taken seriously by American government officials.

Florida Senator Marco Rubio, a vocal critic of the Cuban government and a staunch opponent of normalizing relations with the communist nation, immediately condemned the "harming" of American citizens, noting that there was a long history of Cuban operatives harassing Embassy staff [17]. The episode threatened to derail a 2-year initiative that began under the Obama administration to renew diplomatic ties and normalize relations with the government in Havana. The relationship between Washington and Havana had been frosty ever since the Cold War. Later that same day, Cuban officials issued a strongly worded denial of any involvement in the attacks. "The Ministry categorically emphasizes that Cuba has never, nor would it ever, allow that the Cuban territory be used for any action against accredited diplomatic agents or their families, without exception." It noted that they were first informed of the "alleged incidents" on February 17 of 2017 and that they were distressed that Cuban diplomats were kicked out of the US over the affair. Cuban authorities emphasized that they were keen to cooperate with the United States over the claims as they had nothing to hide [18].

At this point, neither Dorsey nor Nauert had made any reference to a sonic attack. The first public mention of this occurred that very evening when the Associated Press reported on information gleaned from State Department sources who spoke on the condition of anonymity as they were not authorized to speak on the matter publicly. Under the headline: "Hearing Loss of US Diplomats in Cuba Blamed on Covert Device," the report stated that there had been "a string of bizarre incidents that left a group of American diplomats in Havana with severe hearing loss attributed to a covert sonic device." The sources said that after an investigation spanning several months, government officials had "concluded that the diplomats had been exposed to an advanced device that operated outside the range of audible sound and had been deployed either inside or outside their residences. It was not immediately clear if the device was a weapon used in a deliberate attack, or had some other purpose" [19]. This immediately created another mystery: if it was outside the range of human hearing, what were Embassy staff listening to? Over the next several months, the episode remained in the public eye as State Department officials continued to leak information to the media about what was happening behind the scenes, particularly through the Associated Press.

On September 14, the State Department began to refer to what had previously been described as "incidents," with terms like "health attacks," and later, a "crime" [20]. The next day, five members of the Senate Intelligence Committee wrote an urgent letter to President Trump, calling for the expulsion of all Cuban diplomats in the US and closure of the American Embassy in Cuba unless the "attacks" stopped. The senators underscored the seriousness of the situation, noting that they had "caused permanent hearing damage and other significant injuries" [21]. By mid-October, President Trump further stoked tensions between the two countries by proclaiming: "I do believe Cuba is responsible" for the "attack" [22]. White House Chief of Staff John Kelly echoed these sentiments: "We believe that the Cuban government could stop the attacks on our diplomats," he said [23].

Conspicuously, neither Trump, Kelly, nor the senators were able to provide any concrete evidence of an attack or the use of a sonic device. By January 2018, Secretary of State Rex Tillerson was using the term "deliberate attacks," and asserting: "I still believe that the Cuban government…can bring this to an end" [24]. In early September, the head of an American task force looking into the incident, former Libyan Ambassador Peter Bodde, would tell members of the House Foreign Affairs Committee that the State Department had concluded that what happened to both the Americans and Cubans were "attacks." Despite this determination, his assessment of the situation was less than convincing, later telling the hearing: "Let me be clear, the Department does not currently know the mechanism for the cause of the injuries, the source, or the motive behind the attacks in Cuba or when they actually commenced" [25, p 10]. State Department official Kenneth Merten also agreed that it was an attack, yet he noted that "the investigation into the health attacks is ongoing" and there was "much we do not know, including who or what is behind the injuries to our colleagues" [25, p 9]. This begs the question: given the lack of definitive evidence, how could the State Department be so certain that they were attacks? Merten, the former Ambassador to Croatia and Haiti, would later make a curious observation: "I think the State Department and Secretary Tillerson have come to the belief that what happened in Cuba is an attack, because all the information we have seen is that it seems to be targeted specifically at our Embassy and one other Embassy that we know of, Canada's, employees, diplomats" [25, p 46]. This feature is a telltale sign of mass hysteria because it typically follows social networks. In school outbreaks, for instance, it is not uncommon for dozens – even hundreds of students to be affected but not a single teacher, or for children to succumb but no adults, or certain ethnic groups to be stricken in Asian factories, but few if any in others; or even line workers but no managers. The word "attack" was used in the hearing 27 times. Witness after witness used the word, taking the State Department's lead, that is, until it came to Brian Mazanec of the Accountability Office. His written testimony stood out for the use of the word "incident." When pressed by one of the committee members to clarify if what he meant was an "incident" or "attack," it became clear that he was not convinced there had been an attack, and he refused to tow the State Department line: "Sir, we deferred and used the language that the State Department did in our report. But I think this issue emphasizes the importance of the Department addressing some of the communication challenges we identified so they can make these determinations as promptly as possible" [25, p 46]. Two months later White House National Security Advisor John Bolton, known for his hard line with foreign adversaries, would call for tough action on what he assumed was a deliberate attack on US personnel. "I think it's very important that somebody must be held accountable for what happened to our diplomats. It's a fundamental principle of how America operates in the world, that Americans abroad do not get harmed with impunity," he said [26].

In the waning months of 2017, more information about the 'attacks' would be revealed at State Department press briefings and from media leaks, including the revelation that in early November 2016, shortly after the election of President Trump, a small number of workers at the US Embassy in Havana began to experience symptoms that were accompanied by the presence of mysterious high-pitched sounds. The incidents were not officially identified as a health issue until mid-February 2017, at which time the State Department notified the Cuban government in Havana, putting them on notice that the US was aware of the 'acoustical attacks,' and that they needed to stop immediately. None of the 'attacks' occurred at the Embassy, but cither in the residences of the workers which were scattered across the city or in one of two prominent hotels: the Capri and Hotel Nacional de Cuba (National Hotel of Cuba). Several Canadian Embassy staff reported similar experiences, with the Associated Press revealing that they had been contacted by "roughly three dozen" American tourists who had reported hearing strange sounds and feeling unwell while visiting Cuba in recent years [14, 27]. Such reports should not come as a surprise given that the two hotels in question have a combined 646 rooms and at least 34 suites. On any given day, with so many guests, a small number of people are going to be feeling unwell, while there are always going to be ambiguous background noises.

Ever-Increasing Circles

In mid-October 2017, the State Department expelled fifteen more Cuban diplomats in response to the ongoing 'attacks' [28]. By late November, CBS News uncovered information that 2 months earlier, a US Embassy worker in Tashkent, Uzbekistan was evacuated along with his wife after they reported feeling unwell with symptoms similar to what had been described in Cuba. The health incidents coincided with the presence of a high-pitched sound [29]. The pair were reportedly flown out by the State Department for evaluation in the US as senior security officials raised concerns that the Russians may also have been involved in the Cuban attacks since they had a growing influence in Havana. A foreign policy professor at American University, William Leogrande said: "The Russians have been rebuilding their relationship [with Cuba], it deteriorated dramatically after the end of the Cold War. They have a strong presence in Cuba and a historic relationship with Cuban intelligence that might give them the kind of freedom to operate that would provide an opportunity" [29]. State Department spokesperson Heather Nauert later refuted the report, saying, "We can confirm that there was no incident in Uzbekistan" [29].

In June 2018, the *New York Times* reported that a diplomat at a consulate in Guangzhou, China had developed symptoms almost identical to those reported by diplomats in Havana [30]. The man reported experiencing "abnormal sensations of sound and pressure" from late 2017 to April 2018, when he was evacuated to the US for further evaluation. The State Department concluded after a comprehensive assessment (presumably at the University of Pennsylvania) that the diplomat had suffered a mild traumatic brain injury [31]. Several other staff at the Guangzhou consulate were being evacuated for "further evaluation" [31]. The following month, the State Department issued a health alert to US citizens in China, asking them to report any "unusual acute auditory or sensory phenomena" but they denied being aware of any other similar cases in China at the time [31]. Mark Lenzi, a security engineer at the Guangzhou consulate, disputed this claim. He lived in the same complex as the consulate worker who had been evacuated in April and said he had been hearing sounds like "marbles bouncing and hitting a floor" for the past year [31]. He and his family developed a variety of symptoms after hearing the sounds including excruciating headaches and sleeplessness. Lenzi and his family were later evacuated. He criticized the April health alert for giving the impression that only one person was affected. "They knew full well it wasn't," he said [31]. By the end of June 2018, the US State Department had evacuated at least 11 Americans from China, 8 from the consulate in Guangzhou, 1 from the consulate in Shanghai, and 2 from the embassy in Beijing [32]. Details on the Shanghai and Beijing evacuees were sketchy, but the State Department indicated they were being sent to the United States for further evaluation based on preliminary examinations. Secretary of State Mike Pompeo raised the issue with his Chinese counterpart, Wang Yi, in a telephone call and senior State Department officials flew to China to further investigate the problem [32]. Pompeo appointed a committee to review "unexplained health incidents" affecting American diplomats and employees abroad with Deputy Secretary of State, John J. Sullivan, leading the review, assisted by representatives from the Department of Health and Human Services and the Justice Department. Officials admitted that they were "flummoxed" [32]. Complicating matters further, the State Department reported that another American at the embassy in Havana was found to have a "brain injury" from a "sonic attack" bringing the total to 25, and another was being evaluated for brain injury [32]. Press reports were now using the term "brain injury" or "brain trauma" to describe the disorder as though it was a conclusive finding. During a September 2018 conference call sponsored by the Pentagon, Dr. Michael Hoffer from the University of Miami suggested that embassy staff from several other countries may have also been attacked. "Great Britain, Germany, Canada and France described it potentially being present in their embassy individuals," he said. "But we either can't say, or are not allowed to say if we saw any of those individuals" [33]. The spread of similar symptoms to diplomats at Embassies in other parts of the world is significant. The United States has nearly 300 embassies, consulates and diplomatic missions across the globe with thousands of staff who were now on the lookout for strange sounds and vague feelings of unwellness. This is a classic setup for future outbreaks of mass hysteria or sporadic instances of the nocebo effect.

The Alarming Discovery of White Matter Changes

In early December 2017, the Associated Press broke a bombshell story about the 'attacks' in Cuba. Reporter Josh Lederman revealed that doctors treating the victims had uncovered changes in their brains. "Medical testing has revealed the embassy workers developed changes to the white matter tracts that let different parts of the brain communicate, several U.S. officials said, describing a growing consensus held by university and government physicians researching the attacks. White matter acts like information highways between brain cells." Lederman went on to write that "Doctors still don't know how victims ended up with the white matter changes, nor how exactly those changes might relate to their symptoms. U.S. officials wouldn't say whether the changes were found in all 21 patients." This news was dramatic and ominous, and raised more questions than answers. For instance, Dr. Elisa Konofagou, Professor of Biomedical Engineering at Columbia University, was incredulous, pointing out that there is no known association between sound waves affecting white matter tracts. "I would be very surprised," she said, adding that ultrasound in the brain is used frequently in modern medicine, yet physicians "never see white matter tract problems" [34]. Ultrasound is routinely used to image something as delicate as a fetus in the womb, without any known health impacts. The discovery of white matter tract changes made headlines around the world. The *Washington Post* carried the headline: "How bizarre events in Cuba changed embassy workers' brains: U.S. embassy workers woke in the night to strange hums or chirping, and some experienced physical changes in the brain" [35]. The *Philadelphia Inquirer* reported: "Doctors Find Brain Abnormalities in Victims of Cuba Mystery" [36]. *The NBC Today Show* broke the news by reporting that there was "alarming new information this morning about those mysterious invisible attacks on U.S. diplomats in Cuba. Doctors treating the victims who were based at the U.S. Embassy there, have found abnormalities in the white matter of their brains. That tissue helps different parts of the brain communicate with each other. This is the most specific finding so far about physical damage caused by those sonic attacks" [37]. *The Asia News Monitor* in Bangkok reported on the news of the white matter changes along with Secretary of State Rex Tillerson's views that the health impact on the Embassy workers were "targeted attacks" [38]. In London, a journalist for the *Daily Telegraph* wrote that the white matter tract changes to the brains of Embassy staff had left them "permanently damaged" [39].

Skepticism

Soon after the appearance of leaked media reports about the sonic attacks, many experts in physics and acoustics expressed extreme skepticism as they could not fathom how such a device would have worked. They were baffled as to how diplomatic staff situated deep within a hotel or in the confines of a house, could be targeted. Human hearing ranges between approximately 20 and 20,000 Hertz (Hz). Sounds below 20 Hz are known as infrasound, from the word *infra* which is Latin for 'below.' These sounds have been difficult to weaponize due to the inability to focus the wavelengths. The main effect on human health is irritation. Sounds at the high end of the spectrum of human hearing is ultrasound, from the Latin 'beyond.' These sound waves are equally difficult to control as they dissipate rapidly as they travel. Even if the sound waves were to reach a building in an effort to target people inside, most of the waves would bounce harmlessly off the walls before reaching their target. Timothy Leighton, professor of Ultrasonics and Acoustics at Southampton University in the United Kingdom, labeled the claims as Buck Rogers-style science fiction. "If you're talking about a ray-gun rifle knocking out someone with ultrasound…that's not going to happen," he said [40]. A prominent figure in the study of acoustics, Leighton has investigated several claims of ultrasonic exposure and says he has yet to find evidence of an ultrasonic attack. He is skeptical of the Cuban attack claims [41]. Former CIA officer Fulton Armstrong supports Leighton's assessment: "No one has a device that could do this" as "no such device exists," he said [42]. If the claims of a super-sophisticated Russian military weapon were true, and it was possible to focus a wave of energy on a specific victim from a distance with great accuracy to cause illness or incapacitation, why wasn't such a device used on the battlefield to save lives and avoid house-to-house combat in war zones such as Syria and Iraq?

Acoustical experts pointed out other conundrums: most notably that claims of a sonic attack appeared to contravene the laws of physics as sound cannot cause concussions. German physicist and acoustics expert Jürgen Altmann told the *New York Times*: "I know of no acoustic effect that can cause concussion symptoms. Sound going through the air cannot shake your head" [40]. Former MIT acoustics researcher Joseph Pompei was equally incredulous. "Brain damage and concussions, it's not possible," he said, noting that to produce such an effect "Somebody would have to submerge their head into a pool lined with very powerful ultrasound transducers" [43]. A former professor of Neuroscience at Brown University, Seth Horowitz viewed the claims as fanciful. "There isn't an acoustic phenomenon in the world that would cause those type of symptoms" [44]. He observed that while infrasonic sound waves can cause nausea, they would not affect human hearing as "there are no acoustic devices that can cause sudden onset hearing loss that the people involved could not hear" [45].

Acoustic weapons do work and have been used on numerous occasions by governments around the world to control people – it's called loud noise. The sound is annoying and can even be painful but typically there are no long-term effects. Police departments in major cities such as New York, have successfully used Long Range Acoustic Devices or LRADs to disperse crowds of protestors. Dubbed 'sound cannons,' these machines are bulky and conspicuous. In 2015, police in the Philippines blasted Katy Perry music to disperse violent, anti-government protestors [46]. The American Navy has used LRADs to ward off potential attacks by small vessels suspected of carrying explosives, or pirates intent on perpetrating hijackings. The US

Army has even used sound cannons to clear houses of enemy combatants in war zones [47]. The use of sound as a weapon can be found in ancient writings and folklore. The Mandroga plant was said to emit a piercing scream capable of killing a person if its roots were pulled from the ground. A native of the Mediterranean region, it is known today as the Mandrake. The myth surrounding its reputed scream was featured in the Harry Potter film series when sorcerer's apprentices were given earmuffs for protection and taught the proper way to pull them up. The plant's scream was also believed to drive people to insanity [48]. The biblical story of the Battle of Jericho describes the collapse of the city's massive wall after Joshua's army of Israelites marched around the structure blowing trumpets. While this account from the Book of Joshua 6:1–27, is almost certainly mythical, it reveals an age-old human fascination with the potential destructive power of sound. While interest in sound as a weapon continues today, the reputed capabilities of sonic weapons are exaggerated. The internet is rife with grandiose claims touting the quasi-magical powers of covert sonic weapons that range from frying human organs to inducing insanity. Yet, the reality is very different because any such device must conform to the laws of physics, which are not conducive to the development of an effective device in the first place. One of the most comprehensive assessments of acoustical devices was undertaken at the US Air Force Research Laboratory in San Antonio, Texas. Their conclusion: it is "unlikely that high-intensity acoustic energy in the audible, infrasonic, or ultrasonic low-frequency range can provide a device suitable for use as a nonlethal weapon." As a result, research on acoustic weapons has waned as they are widely seen as a waste of research funds and researcher time [49, p 182].

December 2017: The Cuban Sonic Investigation Committee Findings

Soon after US officials first informed the Cubans of the sonic attack "incidents" on February 17, 2017, and the government in Havana was being accused of involvement, they reacted aggressively, concerned that the escalating row might put a damper on the recent warming in diplomatic ties. By March, the Cuban government formed a committee of the country's top scientists to examine the claims and issue a report. They even took the unprecedented step of inviting the Federal Bureau of Investigation to visit the country and conduct their own inquiry – a move that would have been deemed unthinkable during the Cold War. In early December, the Committee announced their findings: there was no evidence of an attack. The panel concluded that the most likely explanation was "collective psychogenic disorder." The probe was thorough and included an examination of the rooms in the two hotels where the diplomats were visiting when they reported their symptoms. Investigators went so far as to canvass neighborhoods where the homes of the affected staff members were located and interviewed about 300 residents. None had reported any health issues associated with unusual sounds. Air and soil samples were analyzed, and the possibility of toxic chemicals was considered and eliminated. Even before the report was issued, the head of the Criminal Division of the Ministry of the

Interior, Lt. Colonel Jorge Alazo said that no tangible cause could be identified. "We've been unable to find anything to prove this situation exists or ever existed," he said. The Ministry's Chief of Diplomatic Security, Colonel Ramiro Ramirez told NBC News that their investigation involved nearly 2000 people, among them "law enforcement agents and the best scientists in our country" [50].

In their report, the panel of scientists addressed the issue of audio recordings that were heard during the 'attacks.' On October 14, 2017, the Associated Press announced that they had obtained a recording of a 'sonic attack' from an Embassy worker. The recording was the first to be released to the public [51]. While the AP could not identify the sound, their description of the recording made it appear to be complex and mysterious. "The sound seemed to manifest in pulses of varying lengths – 7 seconds, 12 seconds, 2 seconds – with some sustained periods of several minutes or more. Then there would be silence for a second, or 13 seconds, or 4 seconds, before the sound abruptly started again… A closer examination of one recording reveals it's not just a single sound. Roughly 20 or more different frequencies, or pitches, are embedded in it, the AP discovered using a spectrum analyzer, which measures a signal's frequency and amplitude." The AP report also noted that "To the ear, the multiple frequencies can sound a bit like dissonant keys on a piano being struck all at once. Plotted on a graph, the Havana sound forms a series of 'peaks' that jump up from a baseline, like spikes or fingers on a hand" [51]. The authors of the AP report then asked an acoustics expert at George Washington University, Kausik Sarkar, to review the recording. "There are about 20 peaks, and they seem to be equally spaced. All these peaks correspond to a different frequency," he said [51]. In January 2019, Biologists Alexander Stubbs of the University of California and Fernando Montealegre-Zapata of Lincoln University in the United Kingdom analyzed the AP 'sonic attack' recording. They found that it was virtually identical to the mating call of the Indies short-tailed cricket (*Anurogryllus celerinictus*) [52]. "No other known continuously calling cricket has a wing stroke rate of 180 per second," Stubbs said, positively identifying the culprit [53]. Short-tailed crickets are known for their tremendous volume, prompting Stubbs to observe that once while recording their mating songs in nearby Central America, he was surprised by the noise they were able to generate. "You can hear them from inside a diesel truck going 40 miles an hour on the highway," he said [54].

The journalists who wrote the original AP story that included an analysis of the 'sonic attack' recording, John Lederman and Michael Weissenstein, made an ironic observation in the opening line of their article: "It sounds sort of like a mass of crickets. A high-pitched whine, but from what?" [51]. US officials provided the Cuban Committee with sound recordings made by diplomats and their family members in and near their homes. Dr. Carlos Barcelo Pérez, an environmental physicist serving on the Cuban Committee, compared these sounds with his own recordings made near the homes of the affected diplomats. When he did, he made an interesting discovery: the frequency of the high-pitched grating sound from the recording given to them from the Americans was at the same frequency as recordings of *Gryllus assimilis* – more commonly known as the Jamaican Field Cricket. This led him to conclude that some of the noises attributed to the 'sonic attack' were chirping crickets, which are capable of producing a loud, metallic sound. Some of his recordings measured the chirping as high as 74.6 decibels [55]. Reaction to the report by the Cuban panel was mixed: some viewed it as government propaganda from a puppet committee. Dr. Alex Berezow, a microbiologist and Senior Fellow of Biomedical Science at the American Council on Science and Health, was outraged by the panel's conclusions. He took exception to their finding that the symptoms were psychological in nature, noting that "hearing loss and brain damage" were not psychogenic symptoms. He wrote that the Cuban government was "playing us for fools" and described the report as "insultingly stupid" [56]. However, the power of expectation can easily fool people. In June 2017, during the Embassy scare, he said he was at home when he heard a mysterious sound that "was so loud and metallic, my brain literally hurt." He contacted an embassy security officer who went out and recorded it. But his housekeeper instantly knew the sound: a Jamaican field cricket. Another diplomat who heard a similar sound described it "as eerie." She said it was "A really nasty sound…very unpleasant." After hearing it on numerous occasions, she came to the realization that it had to be crickets. As the scare went on, she observed that Embassy staff were divided into two broad camps: "the true believers" versus those who were skeptical of an attack [57].

The case took another interesting twist when an American biologist specializing in Latin American cicadas, Allen Sanborn of Barry University in Florida, reported that four FBI agents interviewed him at his home and asked about the possible role of the insects in 'Havana Syndrome.' They played about a dozen recordings made by American diplomatic staff in Havana – sounds that were believed at the time they heard them, to have been part of a sonic attack. While the recordings were not of high quality, he offered the agents his assessment, narrowing it down to three suspects: "crickets, cicadas and katydids," with the Number One suspect being cicadas. As for the possibility that cicadas could cause ear injuries to the diplomats, his answer was an unequivocal 'No.' Based on his 30 years of studying the cicada population in the region, he noted that while they could reach a maximum of 95 decibels, they would have to be shoved into your ear canal to be able to cause any damage whatsoever. He noted that to reach 95 decibels, it would have to be within 20 inches of the person – and even then it would not cause damage [58].

Is it really possible that Americans living in Cuba, many of whom would have grown up listening to the constant chirping of crickets and the whine of cicadas during the summer, did not recognize the sounds of these insects? The answer is 'Yes.' Similar mistakes have occurred many times in the annals of mass psychogenic illness and during social panics where a small group or community believe they are under threat from a hostile agent. A classic example is a case that sociologists refer to as "the Seattle Windshield-pitting epidemic" of 1954. In March, a rumor spread across parts of Washington state, that someone was firing a BB-gun at car windshields. The 'attacks' began in Bellingham, in northwest Washington, and quickly spread. Reports of the "elusive BB-snipers" soon spread the Metropolitan city of Seattle, causing alarm. Oddly, police had no suspects or tangible evidence. During this same period, a second rumor began to circulate – in the wake of widely publicized reports of American Atomic bomb testing in the Pacific

Ocean, it was said some of the radioactive fallout had appeared in Washington State and was falling from the skies, pitting windshields. The scare reached such proportions that by April 15, the Mayor of Seattle contacted President Dwight Eisenhower to seek emergency assistance. Many residents now noticed that there were tiny pit marks, along with small black spheres on their windshields. An investigation by the Environmental Research Laboratory at the University of Washington identified the tiny particles as cenospheres produced by the incomplete combustion of coal. These particles were an ever-present part of everyday life in the region. They could not cause windshield pits. It was concluded that in the wake of the publicity about 'BB-attacks' and the threat from radioactivity, residents began to look at their windshields instead of through them. In doing so, they began to notice the spheres of soot that they would ordinarily have overlooked, and mundane nicks and scratches that are to be found on all windshields, as coming from a phantom BB-sniper or radioactivity [59].

The power of suggestion should not be underestimated. One of the best-known examples of this occurred on the evening of October 30, 1938, when actor Orson Welles produced a radio drama that was broadcast across the United States. As a result, an estimated 1.3–1.7 million listeners in the US and Canada were frightened, a small portion of which panicked and attempted to flee and take shelter. The drama described Martians on towering tripods advancing on parts of New Jersey and New York City [60]. The *New York Times* reported that in a single block in New Jersey, more than 20 families fled their homes to escape the Martian "gas raids," masking their faces with wet handkerchiefs to protect themselves from the "poison gas" [61]. During the imaginary attack, some listeners became convinced that they could feel the heat rays and smell the poison gas as described on the radio, while another began choking from the non-existent fumes [60]. Others said they could hear the "swish" sound of the Martians and the "machine gun fire" in the distance [62] Five students at Brevard College in North Carolina fainted after hearing news of the 'invasion' as "panic gripped the campus for a half hour with many students fighting for telephones to ask their parents to come and get them" [63]. Nerves were especially frayed in Concrete, Washington (population 1000), when a thunderstorm knocked out power during the broadcast, prompting some residents to load their families into cars and head into the mountains. Women reportedly fainted during the incident [64].

In Hamilton, New Jersey, a woman, her voice trembling with fear, told police that she had stuffed wet rags and papers into the crevasses of her doors and windows but it was futile as the fumes were seeping in [65]. Several residents told police that they could see "Martians on their giant machines poised on the Jersey Palisades" – a line of steep cliffs on the lower Hudson River [66, p 379]. At the supposed Martian landing site of Grovers Mill, New Jersey, residents had taken up arms and opened fire at a vague outline barely visible through the fog, punching several holes in the water tower [67, p 5]. A Boston woman was adamant that she could "see the fire" as described on the radio [63]. One man climbed atop a roof and told Bronx police that he "could see the smoke from the bombs, drifting over toward New York. What shall I do?" [68]. In the excitement, some listeners created events that never happened, underscoring the subjective nature of human memory reconstruction. In one case, a devoutly religious woman later recalled that the most realistic part of the broadcast was "the sheet of flame that swept over the entire country. That is just the way I pictured the end" [60, p 181]. There was no mention of any sheet of flame. Some listeners who had tuned into the broadcast in its entirety said they had never heard the disclaimers. The broadcast contained no less than four disclaimers. Just how strong are the nocebo effect and the power of suggestion? A 1998 incident at a California Middle school provides a poignant example. On September 23, three fourth-graders unintentionally swallowed what turned out to be the powerful hallucinogenic drug LSD. They were rushed to a nearby hospital where they would eventually recover. Amid a spate of media reports about the incident, that same day 11 other students at the school recalled having sampled a white powder from a vial. The students believed that they had also ingested LSD and were taken to the hospital suffering from violent outbursts and hallucinations. It was later determined that the powder was harmless. The students quickly recovered and were released within a few hours [69].

References

1. Thomas WI. The child in America. New York: Alfred Knopf; 1932. p. 572.
2. Vergano D. The US government botched its investigation into the mysterious 'sonic attack' in Cuba, emails reveal. BuzzFeed News. 29 May 2019.
3. Nauert H. US Department of State press briefing. Washington, DC. 28 Sept 2017.
4. Wilkinson T. Did covert spy gear cause U.S. and Canadian diplomats in Cuba to lose their hearing? Los Angeles Times Online. 10 Aug 2017.
5. Swanson R, Hampton S, Green-McKenzie J, Diaz-Arrastia R, Grady M, Ragini V, et al. Neurological manifestations among US government personnel reporting directional audible and sensory phenomena in Havana, Cuba. JAMA. 2018;319(11):1125–33. https://doi.org/10.1001/jama.2018.1742.
6. Wilkinson T. The mystery of 'sonic' attacks in Cuba deepens; U.S. diplomats suffered brain injuries… Los Angeles Times. 20 Feb 2018;Sect. A:2.
7. DeYoung K. Neurological injuries found in U.S. staff in Cuba. The Washington Post. 15 Feb 2018;Sect. A:15.
8. Matthew L. Cuba denies role in 'sonic attacks' that left U.S. diplomats with brain damage. Time. 19 Sept 2017. p. 79.
9. Leonard T. Damning evidence. Daily Mail (London). 22 Sept 2017.
10. Finnegan C. Stunning new details in first medical report on US personnel in Cuba. ABC News (American Broadcasting Company, New York). 14 Feb 2018.
11. Stone J. The bare essentials: functional symptoms in neurology. Neurol Pract. 2009;9:179–89. https://doi.org/10.1136/jnnp.2009.177204.
12. Hitt J. Hear no evil. Vanity Fair. 2019;61(2):48. https://www.vanityfair.com/news/2019/01/the-real-story-behind-the-havana-embassy-mystery. Accessed 22 Oct 2019
13. Entous A, Anderson JL. Havana syndrome. The New Yorker. 2018;94(37):34–47. On September 11, 2018, one of the State Department employees who was sent home from Havana, contacted Robert Bartholomew. In a subsequent interview on January 3, 2019, they related the information about *The New Yorker* piece, and told him: "A number of us are similarly skeptical and frustrated by the main scientists and doctors with whom State has been working, and by their failure to explore thoroughly, seriously, the possibility of mass psychogenic illness. Their reasons for discounting it as a possibility are not founded in fact." While they were not one of the patients in the *JAMA* study, they expressed concern with claims that some staff were

unaware that others were hearing sounds and feeling unwell and observed that "we all knew intimate details about each others' issues."

14. Lederman J. US tourist fears he was hit in Cuba, years before diplomats. The Associated Press. 19 Oct 2017.
15. Jenks S. What really happened? The secret sonic war. Podcast created on 2018 Sept 27. https:// www.stitcher.com/podcast/what-really happened/e/56431028?autoplay=true. Accessed 23 June 2019.
16. Nauert H. US Department of State press briefing. Washington, DC. 9 Aug 2017.
17. Rubio M. Rubio statement on Castro regime harming U.S. diplomats in Cuba. Press release. 9 Aug 2017.
18. Cuban Ministry of Foreign Affairs issues statement addressing allegations by the U.S. Granma (Havana, Cuba). 2017 Aug 9. *Granma* is the official newspaper of the Central Committee of the Cuban Communist Party.
19. Lee M, Weissenstein M. Hearing loss of US diplomats in Cuba blamed on covert device. The Washington Post. 9 Aug 2017.
20. Nauert H. US Department of State Press Briefing. 14 Sept and 4 Oct 2017.
21. Rubio M. Rubio, colleagues ask Tillerson to expel Cubans, close embassy after attacks on U.S. diplomats. Press release. 15 Sept 2017.
22. Blitzer W. Trump and McConnell news conference. CNN News airing between 2 and 2:30 p.m. ET. 16 Oct 2017.
23. Cuba could stop 'attacks' against Americans: white house. Reuters. 13 Oct 2017.
24. Lederman J, Lee M. Tillerson says Cuba still risky, but FBI doubts sonic attack occurred. Savannah Morning News (GA). 9 Jan 2018. p. 5.
25. U.S. Policy Toward Cuba, Hearing before the Subcommittee on the Western Hemisphere of the Committee on Foreign Affairs, House of Representatives, 115th Congress, Second Session. 6 Sept 2018.
26. Torres N. Bolton: somebody must be held accountable in Cuba attacks. Miami Herald. 1 Nov 2018.
27. Lederman J. US: a few visitors to Cuba claim symptoms similar to attacks. The Associated Press News. 6 Oct 2017.
28. Attacks on U.S. diplomats in Cuba: response and oversight. US Senate Committee on Foreign Relations, Subcommittee on Western Hemisphere, Transnational Crime, Civilian Security, Democracy, Human Rights, and Global Women's Issues. Attacks on US diplomats in Cuba. Video of the complete hearing published 2018 Jan 9. https://www.foreign.senate.gov/hearings/attacks-on-us-diplomats-in -cuba-response-and-oversight-010918. Accessed 22 July 2019.
29. Dorsey S. Uzbekistan incident raises suspicions of Russian involvement in Cuba attacks. CBS News. 28 Nov 2017.
30. Harris G. 25th person at U.S. embassy in Cuba is mysteriously sickened. The New York Times. 21 June 2018.
31. Kuo L. 'Sonic attack' fears as more US diplomats fall ill in China. The Guardian. 7 June 2018.
32. Myers SL. More Americans evacuated from China over mysterious ailments. The New York Times. 30 June 2018.
33. Weinberger S. Scientists say 'neuroweapons' were behind Cuba attacks. Yahoo News. 10 Sept 2018.
34. Brain abnormalities found in victims of US embassy attack in Cuba. The Guardian. 6 Dec 2017.
35. Selk A. How bizarre events in Cuba changed embassy workers' brains: U.S. embassy workers woke in the night to strange hums or chirping, and some experienced physical changes in the brain. The Washington Post Blog. 6 Dec 2017.
36. Doctors find brain abnormalities in victims of Cuba mystery. Philadelphia Inquirer. 10 Dec 2017. p. 9.
37. Guthrie S. NBC News Today. 6 Dec 2017.

38. Cuba: Tillerson says diplomatic people in Cuba were 'targeted.' Asia News Monitor (Bangkok, Thailand). 8 Dec 2017.
39. Embassy staff in Cuba left with brain injuries: world bulletin. The Daily Telegraph. 7 Dec 2017. p. 15.
40. Zimmer C. A 'sonic attack' on diplomats in Cuba? These scientists doubt it. The New York Times. 5 Oct 2017.
41. Sonic weapons evidence far from sound following 'attacks' in Cuba and China. University of Southampton press release. 20 June 2018.
42. Kornbluh P. Trump's non-sonic attack on Cuba. The Nation. 5 Oct 2017.
43. Lederman J, Weissenstein M, Lee M. Cuba mystery grows: new details on what befell US diplomats. The Chicago Tribune. 15 Sept 2017.
44. Loria K. US diplomats returned from Cuba with brain injuries and hearing loss, and mysterious 'sonic weapons' could be to blame. Business Insider Australia. 16 Sept 2017.
45. Gearan A. U.S. investigating whether American diplomats were victims of sonic attack in Cuba. The Washington Post. 10 Aug 2017.
46. Felipe C. Katy Perry roar at anti-APEC rallyists. The Philippine Star. 20 Nov 2015.
47. Evers M. The weapon of sound: sonic canon gives pirates an earful. Der Spiegel. 2015 Nov 15. https://www.spiegel.de/international/spiegel/the-weapon-of-sound-sonic-canon-gives-pirates-an-earful-a-385048.html. Accessed 22 Oct 2019.
48. Clark H. The mandrake fiend. Folklore. 1962;73(4):257–69.
49. Jauchem J. High-intensity acoustics for military nonlethal applications. Mil Med. 2007;72:182–9.
50. Mitchell A, Murray M, Abou-Sabe K. Cubans forcefully reject blame for U.S, diplomats' mystery ailments. NBC News. 2017 Oct 25. https://www.nbcnews.com/news/us-news/cubans-forcefully-reject-blame-u-s-diplomats-mystery-ailments-n813581. Accessed 15 Oct 2019.
51. Lederman J, Weissenstein M. Dangerous sound? What Americans heard in Cuba attacks? The Associated Press. 13 Oct 2017.
52. Stubbs A, Montealegre-Zapata F. Recording of 'sonic attacks' on U.S. diplomats in Cuba spectrally matches the echoing call of a Caribbean cricket. bioRxiv 510834; doi: https://doi.org/10.1101/510834. Researchers identified six separate independent lines of evidence to support their conclusions including 1) a carrier frequency of 7 kHz; 2) the pulse repetition rate of 180 Hz; 3) the timescale and degree of pulse repetition instability; 4) the phenomenology of the echo; 5) the number of oscillations per pulse; and 6) the frequency decay of approximately 1 kHz over the pulse duration.
53. Hickey J. Recorded sounds that plagued U.S. diplomats in Cuba just crickets hard at work. Berkeley News. 10 Jan 2019.
54. Zimmer C. The sounds that haunted U.S. diplomats in Cuba? Lovelorn crickets, scientists say. The New York Times. 4 Jan 2019.
55. Stone R. Cuban panel claims stress caused mystery illness. Science. 2017;358(6368):1236–7.
56. Berezow A. Sonic attack: Cuba playing us for fools. American Council on Science and Health News. 2017 Dec 6. https://www.acsh.org/news/2017/12/06/sonic-attack-cuba-playing-us-fools-12245. Accessed 26 Oct 2019.
57. Stone R. Sonic attack or mass paranoia? Science. 2018. https://doi.org/10.1126/science.aau5386.
58. Golden T, Rotella S. The sound and the fury: inside the mystery of the Havana embassy. ProPublica. 2018 Feb 14. https://www.propublica.org/article/diplomats-in-cuba. Accessed 11 Nov 2019.
59. Medalia NZ, Larsen O. Diffusion and belief in a collective delusion. Am Sociol Rev. 1958;23:180–6.
60. Cantril H. The invasion from Mars: a study in the psychology of panic. Princeton (NJ): Princeton University Press; 1947.
61. Radio listeners in panic, taking war drama as fact. The New York Times. 31 Oct 1938. p. 4.

62. Bartholomew RE. Introduction. In: Wells HG, editor. The war of the worlds. New York: Cosimo Classics; 2012:v–ix. See pvi.
63. Scare is nation-wide. The New York Times. 31 Oct 1938. p. 4.
64. Women faint as lights go out at Concrete. Seattle Post-Intelligencer. 31 Oct 1938. p. 1.
65. Terror spread here by hoax. Trenton Evening Times. 31 Oct 1938. p. 2.
66. Markush R. Mental epidemics: a review of the old to prepare for the new. Public Health Rev. 1973;2:353–442.
67. Marvin S. The halloween radio spoof that shook a nation. Parade. 29 Oct 1975. p. 4–5.
68. Radio war drama creates a panic. The New York Times. 31 Oct 1938. p. 4.
69. Moore S, Ramirez M. 3 sickened Pacoima students ingested LSD; 11 others hospitalized 4th graders had no drugs in system. The Los Angeles Times. 25 Sept 1998.

The Crisis Deepens

Or in the night, imagining some fear,
How easy is a bush supposed a bear.

–William Shakespeare [1]

On January 9, 2018, Florida Senator Marco Rubio chaired a special hearing of the Senate Foreign Relations Committee on the "Attacks on U.S. Diplomats in Cuba." It turned into a political spectacle. State Department Medical Director Dr. Charles Rosenfarb was the star witness, proclaiming: "The findings suggest that this is not a case of mass hysteria," although conspicuously, he refused to completely dismiss the possibility, later prefacing: "No cause has been ruled out" [2]. The Hearing ended with Rubio concluding that an attack took place and the Cuban government was either directly or indirectly responsible. Despite these claims, no definitive evidence was presented to prove that Cuba was the source of the 'attacks,' was complicit with a third party – or that an attack had even taken place. Rubio, a long-time opponent of reopening ties with Cuba, appeared to be taking the opportunity to advance his own political agenda. Even before the hearing, a dispute over the nature of the episode had erupted between two senior committee members. While Rubio openly referred to the "incidents" as "attacks," his fellow Republican Senator Jeff Flake of Arizona noted that an FBI investigation still had found "no evidence" that an attack took place, sonic or otherwise [3]. During the hearing, which was supposedly fair and impartial, Rubio asked blatantly leading questions that were clearly intended to ridicule the possibility of psychogenic illness. At one point he asked Rosenfarb if there was "any thought given to the fact that this is a case of mass hysteria. That a bunch of people are just being hypochondriacs and making it up" [2]. This line of questioning was flawed as it implies that victims of mass psychogenic illness are hypochondriacs and fabricators when they are not. Mass hysteria is neither a psychiatric disorder nor a condition that involves feigning illness for some benefit. Victims experience real symptoms and are not faking. Rubio's portrayal of psychogenic illness victims was wrong and reflected antiquated stereotypes which contribute to the present-day stigma that is associated with outbreaks.

© Springer Nature Switzerland AG 2020
R. W. Baloh, R. E. Bartholomew, *Havana Syndrome*,
https://doi.org/10.1007/978-3-030-40746-9_2

Dr. Rosenfarb's testimony stands out for its vagueness, as he noted that the staffers affected described "a multitude of symptoms, many of which are not easily quantifiable and not easily attributable to a specific cause." He said that "the most challenging factor is the lack of certainty about the causative agent and, therefore, the precise mechanism of the injuries suffered" [2]. State Department executive Todd Brown echoed Rosenfarb's sentiments, stating that they first became aware of the "health attacks" in late December 2016. Of particular interest was his statement that "In the early stages of trying to understand what may have been occurring, Post leadership and supporting offices in Washington believed it was likely a form of harassment by forces hostile to the United States and our presence in Cuba" [2]. Another State Department official who testified, Francisco Palmieri, also noted that as soon as they "identified a pattern connecting these unusual events," that is the appearance of mysterious sounds coinciding health problems, by mid-February they assumed that the Cuban government was involved in the episode and they ordered them to stop [2]. Rosenfarb made another curious remark in his testimony: he said that the symptoms occurred *"within minutes to hours of the event"* [2]. In other words, in some cases from the time the mysterious sounds were heard to the time people reported feeling unwell, *hours had passed.* This is a *very broad* time range and an important observation because of the State Department's initial assumption and the first port of call after they became aware of the illness cluster, was the sonic exposure hypothesis. The sounds accompanying the symptoms were the reason that the patients were referred to an otolaryngologist – an ear, nose, and throat specialist with the University of Miami by the name of Dr. Michael Hoffer. The University was a natural fit for the State Department as it was the embassy's evacuation point. He was, as Dr. Rosenfarb described him, "highly experienced in evaluating acoustic injuries in military personnel" [2]. Hoffer had worked previously with veterans of the fighting in Iraq and Afghanistan, who had suffered inner ear trauma.

Between February and April 2017, Hoffer evaluated 80 embassy staff and family members, of which 16 were felt to have a clinical picture consistent with mild traumatic brain injury or concussion. That July, Rosenfarb convened a panel of academic experts to review the clinical material gathered so far and although the panel felt that some of the patient's symptoms might have been due to a variety of causes including even normal aging and stress, the consensus was that the symptoms were most likely due to "trauma from a non-natural source." Considering the parallels with mild traumatic brain injury, the well-known brain injury center at the University of Pennsylvania was chosen to reevaluate the 16 people identified at the University of Miami. In the convening months, 8 additional cases were identified with a similar clinical profile bringing the total to 24, 21 of which were tested and reported in the *Journal of the American Medical Association* study [2].

After the hearing, Arizona Senator Jeff Flake, who had received classified briefings by the FBI on the evidence for a sonic attack – or lack thereof, was openly displeased with the inflammatory rhetoric of his fellow Republican Rubio, telling CNN: "The Cubans bristle at the word 'attack.' I think they are justified at doing so. The FBI has said there is no evidence of an attack. We shouldn't be using that word" [4]. Rubio fired back on Twitter that Flake lacked common sense and was not fully informed.

"It's a documented FACT that 24 U.S. govt officials & spouses were victims of some sort of sophisticated attack while stationed in Havana," he wrote, adding that "It is impossible to conduct 24 separate & sophisticated attacks on US Govt personnel in Havana without #CastroRegime knowing about it" [5]. This prompted the Cuban Ambassador to the US, José Ramón Cabañas, to equate the claims of Cuban involvement to the belief in other dubious phenomena. "It is evident that to attack #Cuba some people don't need any evidence. Next stop UFOs!!," he Tweeted [6].

The State Department's initial reaction to this saga is the equivalent of someone hearing a strange noise in their attic in the middle of the night and immediately assuming it's a ghost and calling in a 'psychic' investigator when they should have called a builder. Their response can be summarized in a single sentence with an old medical adage: 'When you hear the sounds of hoof-beats in the night, first think horses, not zebras.' Instead of initially examining mundane explanations, State Department officials opted for the most exotic hypothesis early on. Instead of looking for horses, they began searching for zebras. Unicorns would be an even more accurate description because however unlikely, the existence of zebras is at least possible, whereas the use of sonic weapons would defy the laws of physics. In short, the US government had created an imaginary assailant, aided and abetted by poor oversight from one of the world's top medical journals. In the seventeenth century Spanish novel, *El Ingenioso Hidalgo Don Quijote de la Mancha* (*The Ingenious Nobleman Don Quixote of La Mancha*) by Miguel de Cervantes (1547–1616), the protagonist Don Quixote comes upon a cluster of windmills and sets off to fight them. "Do you see over yonder, friend Sancho, thirty or forty hulking giants? I intend to do battle with them and slay them. With their spoils we shall begin to be rich for this is a righteous war…" His servant Sancho Panza asks, "What giants?" to which his master responded, "Those you see over there…with their long arms. Some of them have arms well-nigh two leagues in length." Sancho replied: "Those over there are not giants but windmills. Those things that seem to be their arms are sails which, when they are whirled around by the wind, turn the millstone" [7]. In modern times, Don Quixote's reaction has given rise to the phrase, 'Tilting at windmills,' which is now commonly used to refer to people who are attacking imaginary enemies. This is exactly what the US government had done: they initiated a fight with an imaginary enemy of their own creation. As American journalist Walter Lippmann once observed, "under certain conditions men respond as powerfully to fictions as they do to realities, and that in many cases they help to create the very fictions to which they respond. Let him cast the first stone who…never saw a plot, a traitor, or a spy where there was none" [8].

Once the determination was made in early 2017 that the symptoms originated from a sonic device, American diplomats who were being posted to Havana "were quietly warned they could face a mysterious threat that was causing American Foreign Service officers to fall ill, some with long-lasting symptoms" [9]. But these briefings went beyond mere counseling. Those diplomats who were about to be posted to Havana were played audio recordings made by staff in Cuba, of the mysterious sounds that had accompanied their symptoms. These recordings were later identified by experts on insects as crickets and cicadas. These actions encouraged more 'attacks' because new Embassy staff were on the lookout for sounds that resembled these very insects. As one Embassy worker told us: "If, prior to deploying to Havana, a government official were given this recording and told it was the hallmark of a debilitating attack, it is completely understandable that said official would arrive in Havana, hear the insects not long after, and fear the worst" [10]. By counseling future Embassy staff over the perceived threat, an expectation of illness was created, and with it, a frame through which future sounds and symptoms were to be interpreted. Now, what in the past had been a mundane noise, took on a whole new possibility. As a result, new Embassy staff in Cuba came to expect that they and their colleagues were being attacked. As a result, they became hyperaware of sounds in their environment and grew fearful that they were signs of an acoustical attack. This is a classic set-up for an outbreak of mass psychogenic illness and for activating the nocebo effect. The irony of the Committee Hearings is that Marco Rubio, who had been dismissive of the Cuban panel of experts probing the sonic attack claims, presided over what any objective observer would describe as a 'kangaroo court' – a hearing with a predetermined outcome. He was clearly not interested in entertaining psychological explanations for the symptoms.

The *JAMA* Fiasco

In this section, we take a closer look at the February 2018 *JAMA* study that many media outlets latched onto as strong evidence or even proof of an attack or targeted energy exposure. Conducted by investigators at the University of Pennsylvania School of Medicine in Philadelphia, the physicians examined 21 Embassy patients, concluding that every one of them was suffering from concussion-like symptoms [11]. They also dismissed claims that it was a case of mass psychogenic illness. But here is where the story takes a surprising twist: for a study published in one of the world's leading medical journals, it was filled with flaws. The authors made grand claims that were not supported by their own evidence. The first thing that stands out in the article is the manner in which the study was written. It was not presented in a neutral manner. Parts of it read like government propaganda. The biased nature of the study is evident on the very first page as the authors make it sound like it is a fact that there was this unknown energy source causing people to get sick in Cuba. They wrote that the purpose of the study was "to describe the neurological manifestations that followed exposure to an unknown energy source." This was certainly not demonstrated in the article. They should have written that the study's purpose was to describe the neurological manifestations following *the alleged exposure* to an unknown energy source. This is basic science: stay within the limitations of the data.

Another curious aspect of the study are claims about brain trauma; that the patients were suffering from damage to their brains and concussion-like symptoms. They wrote that there was "persistent cognitive, vestibular, and oculomotor dysfunction, as well as sleep impairment and headaches." What does this mean in lay terms? 'Vestibular' refers to the parts of the inner ear that control balance and brain connections. 'Oculomotor function' refers to the control of eye movements.

Problems associated with these brain systems often result in dizziness and imbalance. The neurology team further noted that while there was no history of head trauma, "These individuals appeared to have sustained injury to widespread brain networks." The injuries were so severe that 14 of the 21 patients were still unable to return to work at the time the study was published [11, p 1132]. Despite these assertions, their evidence was far from convincing. Shortly after the Cuban sonic investigation panel issued their skeptical findings in early December 2017, information was leaked to the media by some members of this study, strongly rebuffing the claims. It was reported that MRI scans conducted by physicians at the University of Miami and Pennsylvania revealed white matter tract damage and noted that their findings would soon be published in the *Journal of the American Medical Association* [12]. *When the JAMA study was published in February 2018, it* found "nonspecific white matter changes in some individuals, but were otherwise unrevealing" [13, p 1098]. Of the 21 patients tested, most findings were normal. Only three showed white matter changes: two were mild and one was moderate. White matter tract changes are common in an array of conditions ranging from migraine and depression to normal aging. While media leaks by members of the study team claimed that there were significant changes to white matter in the brains of the patients, their actual data did not live up to the hype. In fact, the findings are what one would expect in a group of 21 people who were randomly selected off the street. As for the other dramatic finding of concussion-like symptoms, two neurologists who examined the study and wrote an accompanying editorial, Christopher Muth and Stephen Lewis, were skeptical, pointing out that many of the symptoms overlap with a host of medical and psychiatric conditions and there were no structural changes to the brain. In short, their evidence was vague and inconclusive [13, p 1099].

Other scientists were not only unconvinced, they were astounded by what was being claimed with little or no supporting evidence. The editor of the respected journal *Cortex*, Dr. Sergio Della Sala of the University of Edinburgh described the study as an example of "poor neuropsychology." He said that the standards for neurological impairment used in the *JAMA* study were so arbitrarily high that it gave rise to many false positives [14]. Della Sala would later observe that based on the standard used, "anybody tested – you, me, the Penn scientists, the JAMA editors, the US Embassy personnel," could be classified as impaired [15]. *By defining impairment as any test score under the 40th percentile of normal responses, 4 out of 10 normal people would qualify as being pathological.* He wrote that using a 40 percent threshold was "unheard of in clinical practice or research," while the 5th percentile would be a more suitable cutoff. In noting that symptoms experienced by diplomats in Cuba have been described as mysterious, Della Sala observed that the real mystery was "how such a poor neuropsychological report could have passed the scrutiny of expert reviewers in a first class outlet" as the *Journal of the American Medical Association* [14, p 388]. In reality, the manuscript submitted by the neurological team at the University of Pennsylvania failed to pass the review process unscathed. Prior to acceptance, in January 2018, one of us (Dr. Baloh) was given the manuscript to review. He recommended rejection and observed that their claims seemed more like science fiction than science, and noted numerous inconsistencies.

For instance, some of the subjects did not hear the sound, and for others that did, it was very brief. Most reported hearing a high-pitched sound but a few described it as low-pitched. The descriptions were all over the place with terms like "humming," "grinding metal," "piercing squeals," and "buzzing." The symptoms were also very broad including fatigue, dizziness, unsteadiness, headache, tinnitus, hypersensitivity to sound, sleep disorders, and cognitive impairment. Most of the subjects were given a battery of eye movement and balance tests, many of which Professor Baloh helped to develop. While the authors claimed to have found indications of brain and ear damage caused by the sounds, the evidence fell short. Dr. Baloh saw a familiar pattern. Every week in his dizziness clinic, he saw several patients with *identical symptoms* including the nonspecific test findings reported by the University of Pennsylvania team. The condition, which is more common than most people realize, is now called Persistent Postural Perceptual Dizziness. This recently described syndrome is a functional disorder of the nervous system featuring dizziness, headaches and balancing problems. The driving factor behind it is stress and anxiety. He told the *JAMA* editors that more details were needed about the sound exposure and patient symptoms.

Symptoms like difficulty concentrating, brain fog, memory problems, and sleep-related complaints such as drowsiness and insomnia, were present in nearly all patients. These complaints are common in people with anxiety, depression and both individual and epidemic forms of psychogenic illnesses. Visual issues such as sensitivity to light, difficulty reading, and eye strain were commonly reported but when tested, there was no visual impairment. Impaired convergence and eye tracking found in about half the patients are *extremely common findings in anxious subjects.* Finally, three-quarters of the patients complained of headaches and about half of these had sensitivity to light and sound. These are typical of migraine headaches. Stress is a well-known trigger of migraine and it is likely that some of these patients had migraines or a genetic susceptibility to migraines, since they affect about 15 percent of the population. The conclusion of the Penn brain trauma specialists that the symptoms and test findings in these embassy staff and family members exposed to a "sonic attack" were similar to those of patients with mild traumatic brain injury, is a classic example of a blind man feeling an elephant from his perspective. The lead author of the *JAMA* article, Dr. Randel Swanson would assert: "If you took any one of these patients and put them into a brain injury clinic, and you didn't know their background, you would think they had a traumatic brain injury from being in a car accident or a blast in the military. It's like a concussion without a concussion" [16]. But what if you put them in a dizziness clinic, a headache clinic, a post-traumatic stress disorder clinic or an anxiety disorder clinic? Would they be diagnosed with persistent postural perceptual dizziness, tension or migraine headaches, PTSD and anxiety disorder? Very likely. The process of referring patients with non-specific symptoms to a clinic specializing in brain trauma can shape the symptoms into a specific pattern. This is a concern because it will prolong recovery time as fear and negative expectations are what elicited the symptoms in the first place. If the patients believe they have brain damage, those negative expectations are likely to continue and delay recovery.

The potential role of bias is also relevant to the events in Cuba. The impact of expectation on symptoms can be powerful. Scientists even have a name for it: confirmation bias. Neurologist Mitchell Valdés-Sosa observes that many of the physicians who were working on the case were exhibiting just such a bias and were not able to make an objective assessment. "So, when you look at all the potential alleged weapons that could have been employed, none of them are possible according to the laws of physics and principles of engineering. And on the other hand, you have no evidence for brain injury and for hearing loss in a large group of subjects; so, the whole case collapses. It's simply a construction that I think has spiralled out of control, based on theories that have been accepted as facts and then these pseudo facts are used to construct other theories…none of which are scientifically sustainable or acceptable" [17, p 16]. Valdés-Sosa makes a strong point because many media outlets and US government officials were fueling the sonic or microwave attack scenario and were making claims that could not be substantiated. When as in this case, doctors have certain preconceived explanations in mind, "the first things that fit with your conceived theory are the ones you use more and the rest you sort of brush under the rug…And in this case, there was a theory from the start: that there were attacks. And then everything that we've seen published and the leaks to the media, all are based on this unconfirmed idea" [17, pp 18–19].

Dismissing Mass Hysteria

One of the most stunning claims in the *JAMA* study was the way they dismissed psychogenic illness, noting that the symptoms in the Embassy staff were prolonged, that a majority of victims were men, and the subjects were cooperative and showed no evidence of faking. These are all common misconceptions and show an alarming lack of familiarity with the topic. Psychogenic illness affects both men and women, and while there is no brain damage, the symptoms are real and can be disabling. Furthermore, when neurological symptoms are involved, they can persist for months, even years. By performing extensive diagnostic testing and raising the possibility of an array of conditions including brain damage, the doctors may have inadvertently prolonged the outbreak. Malingering – the faking of illness or injury for some benefit, has nothing to do with this case. It is the wrong term.

In a later interview, one of the study authors said that the team had discounted a psychological cause as there was no collusion among patients. He said, to have "mass hysteria" you would have to have all of the patients "in collusion together to make sure all their symptoms match" [18]. This assertion is as remarkable as it is untrue. Collusion and mass hysteria are chalk and cheese. They are unrelated. Mass psychogenic illness outbreaks occurring in populations that are under prolonged stress, often feature *neurological symptoms*. The Cuban diplomats were certainly in a hostile environment on foreign soil in a location that was known for closely surveilling and harassing American Embassy staff. The study team also claim that some patients had not heard about the symptoms previously – discounting mass suggestion as a possible cause. This claim stretches credulity given the close-knit nature of the diplomatic staff in Cuba and at other posts around the world. It took an average of 203 days before the patients were interviewed. Memories fade with time and are easily distorted, especially over such a significant period. Furthermore, one Embassy staffer who was evacuated from Havana vehemently challenged claims that some workers were unaware of the attack claims and associated health issues, telling us that not only were Embassy employees all aware of the medical concerns, "we all knew intimate details about each others' issues" [10].

In his review, Dr. Baloh warned of flaws in the methodology and conclusions, cautioning the editor that it would be risky to publish this manuscript in its current form and warning of a likely backlash from the scientific community. It was published anyway – and the reaction from the scientific community was swift. After a torrent of criticism of their conclusions appeared in a subsequent issue of the journal, the study team failed to acknowledge that their study contained any flaws. This prompted the entire editorial board of the respected European-based journal *Cortex*, to take the rare and extraordinary step of calling on the authors of the study to either clarify the methods they had used to arrive at their conclusions or retract the study. They wrote that criticisms of the serious methodological flaws that followed publication of the *JAMA* study was met with an attempt to cover up those flaws. "The authors' surprising response to these criticisms was not to defend or explain the original methods, but to claim that the methods used were in fact different from those stated in the original paper... The two descriptions of the methods, which are both highly questionable, cannot both be true: either what was reported in the original paper is false, or what is stated in the rebuttal is false (or possibly both). ...they cannot yield the same results." They went on to question how it was possible that one of the world's leading medical journals could publish such a flawed study [19, pA1]. As Sergio Della Sala and his colleagues at *Cortex* would later observe, the defense of using the 40th percentile threshold by the authors of the *JAMA* study was so ambiguous as to be incomprehensible [20]. In noting the old Venetian saying: "the mending is worse than the hole," they wrote that the *JAMA* study authors "have tried to patch over an unjustifiable threshold for impairment reported in the original paper with an even less cogent statement of their actual criterion in the rebuttal. Only two things are clear in this murky matter: that the crucial criterion for cognitive impairment was mis-stated in the original paper, and that the neuropsychological data presented do not support the conclusion that whatever happened in Cuba resulted in persistent cognitive decline" [21, p 288].

In defending their original study, the *JAMA* authors also tried to play the 'government secrecy card' with statements like "we must continue to withhold certain sensitive information" and "despite the preliminary nature of the data..." [20]. These are red flags. They are essentially asking us to take their word for it and to trust their judgment. Science does not work this way. Scientists present evidence and draw conclusions based on that evidence, not information that is supposedly being kept hidden from the public. The fact remains that when you take away the dubious claims of white matter track changes, concussion-like symptoms, and hearing loss, we are left with a classic outbreak of mass psychogenic illness. It is also difficult to trust people – even accomplished scientists, when they have made such egregious errors like conflating mass psychogenic illness with collusion and malingering, and claims of brain damage based on the flimsiest of evidence, or using standards of neurological impairment that would classify 40 percent of the population as pathological. The *JAMA* study was a powerful influence on public opinion and reinforced a belief that some type of attack had been perpetrated on Embassy staff. Journalists lapped up the study, with many media outlets downplaying the accompanying editorial and commentary that was sharply critical. Many failed to mention it altogether.

The Golden Investigation

At nearly the same time that the *JAMA* study was published, Pulitzer Prize-winning investigative journalist Tim Golden released the results of his probe into the Cuban affair. He and fellow reporter Sebastian Rotella interviewed over three dozen American and foreign officials and gained access to confidential government documents on the case [22]. In doing so, they managed to piece together the early timeline of events which would prove crucial to understanding how the sonic attack hypothesis evolved. The first two incidents coincided with the death of Fidel Castro on November 25. On or near that date, two undercover intelligence officers who lived in upscale neighborhoods in the western suburbs of Havana would later divulge that they had heard strange high-pitched sounds while in their residences at night but kept their experiences to themselves. Golden reports that it was not until December 30, 2016, that the first undercover officer, a fit man in his thirties, sought medical advice inside the Embassy. He walked into the Embassy staff clinic complaining of headaches, difficulty hearing, and acute pain in one ear. The symptoms were not unlike those treated by physicians every day. They were nothing too alarming or sinister, and certainly nothing to suggest a sonic attack. But he also made an unusual observation: the complaints coincided with what appeared to be "a beam of sound" that "seemed to have been directed at his home." The man's condition was reported to the head of the American diplomatic mission in Havana, Jeffrey DeLaurentis, and the head of diplomatic security, Anthony Spotti. Shortly after, Embassy officials became aware that two other CIA officers working with the Embassy had reported hearing strange sounds while in their homes during the previous month. They would later describe them as "sharp" and "disorienting." Yet at the time, they were not so sharp or disorienting that they had reported it to their superiors or thought they were the subject of an attack. As former CIA agent Fulton Armstrong who once worked undercover in Cuba, would later observe, patient zero "was lobbying, if not coercing, people to report symptoms and to connect the dots" – all within a tightly knit community of Embassy staff who were working in hostile, foreign territory [23].

After initial skepticism senior diplomats and intelligence officials at the Embassy assumed that the incidents were a form of harassment by Cuban operatives who were thought to have been surveilling them. While the operatives were almost certainly being watched, which was normal practice, the evidence that they were being harassed by a sonic device, was flimsy at best. For instance, one of the more con-crete incidents involved the wife of an Embassy employee who reported hearing a strange sound outside their house, only to look out and see a speeding van. This ambiguous event was later viewed as "one of the more significant pieces of circum-stantial information" [22]. On March 29, DeLaurentis summoned all Embassy staff with security clearances and told them that while the situation was fluid and there were many unknowns, they may have been the targets of some type of actions by the Cubans. He encouraged anyone present to contact the Embassy medical section if they suspected that they had been exposed. To avoid panic and the possibility of counterintelligence agents knowing what they knew, it was decided to keep news of the incidents, which were considered classified information, quiet and not mention them to most of the other staff. It was even kept from their families. This generated anger and alarm in some of those present and stoked fear and uncertainty about the possibility that some staff may have been targeted by the Cubans. It was at this point, Golden would write, that health anxieties among Embassy staff and their families, would explode. "Within barely a month, diplomats reported a flurry of new incidents. By the end of April, more than 80 diplomats, family members, and other personnel – a very high proportion for a mission that included about 55 American staff – had asked to be checked out by the Miami medical team" [22]. The impor-tance of his report is that it provides a vital backdrop against which the first few 'attacks' occurred: relatively mundane health complaints and ambiguous reports of sounds. Despite having little concrete information to go on, senior diplomats had concluded that most likely, their staff was being targeted by the Cubans.

By April 2017, officials at the American Embassy in Havana had taken the extreme measure of advising its staff to sleep away from the windows in the middle of a room. This dramatic move was of particular concern for diplomats who were stationed in Havana with young children. As one worker observed, it was a fearful time. "Everybody was in a frenzy about it, they said. "We had a big window in the front of the house. It was a horrible feeling. We just thought, 'Oh my God, we're in harm's way'…You start to feel paranoid" [24]. In late April, Jeffrey DeLaurentis met with the ambassadors of several close allies including France, Britain, and Canada, told them of the 'attacks' and asked if their staff had reported similar expe-riences. By early May, Canadian ambassador Patrick Parisot met with his Cuban diplomatic staff to relay the warning and asked if anyone had been feeling unwell or heard strange noises. As a result, 27 Canadians sought treatment including Embassy employees and their family members who presented with an array of ambiguous symptoms: headaches, nose bleeds, dizziness, insomnia. Some recalled hearing vague noises; many did not [22]. The pattern of illness in the Canadians was differ-ent to the Americans. As a Canadian official noted: "In most cases, there weren't really attacks that we could point to… The American experience was all about acoustic events and people feeling ill, and we had people feeling ill with limited connections to acoustic events" [22]. In any given population, you are going to have people feeling unwell. This explains why at least three dozen American tourists visiting the two Cuba hotels where the attacks had supposedly occurred, also claimed to have felt unwell after hearing a mysterious sound, *but only after being primed by the first news reports of the 'attacks' in August 2017, and most of these 'attacks' had supposedly occurred years earlier.* There is no other plausible explanation for this pattern other than mass psychogenic illness.

Spectacle in Miami

The word 'spectacle' is Latin for "a public show." This aptly describes the events of early December 2018 and the media reaction that would follow in spreading the misleading narrative that the American Embassy workers had all suffered ear damage. When in early 2017, Dr. Michael Hoffer performed the first examinations on the sick diplomats and their family members, he concluded that several had symptoms that were suggestive of mild traumatic brain injury. However, over a year and a half later, on December 12, 2018, when Hoffer and his research team released the results of their study in the journal *Laryngoscope Investigative Otolaryngology,* they drew a completely different conclusion: they said the symptoms were from inner ear damage [25]. He and his colleagues claimed that every one of the 25 Embassy staff that his team had examined had damage to the otolith organs which regulate balance, gravity, and sense of motion. The study focused on 35 people examined at the University of Miami's Miller School of Medicine who were seen between 1 week and 2 months after their most recent exposure. It looked at 25 Embassy staff who reported symptoms and direct exposure to either a noise or pressure sensation, and 10 people who were with a victim at the time of an 'attack,' but did not exhibit symptoms, although "one reported an extremely brief sensation of exposure to a force wave and a second heard a very brief, high-pitched noise for a few seconds on a single occasion" [25, p 3]. Those affected said that the sound was localized and capable of following them around the room; several reported that the noise immediately stopped if they opened a door and went outside. The most common symptom was dizziness (92 percent), followed by cognitive problems like difficulty concentrating, forgetfulness, taking longer to process information, and being in a mental fog (56 percent). Hearing loss and tinnitus were reported in 32 percent of subjects, ear pain (28 percent), and headache (24 percent).

Dr. Hoffer told a press conference that was called to announce the results of the study: "This is objective…It's not controversial. The evidence is there. The people had abnormalities" [26]. In commenting on the significance of the study, Dr. Henri Ford, Dean of the Miller School, observed: "This is a perfect example of how academic medicine brings together expertise and collaboration in the name of discovery and science" [27]. In response to the study, *U.S. News & World Report* proclaimed: "U.S. Diplomats Show Inner-Ear Damage After Mysterious Sonic Attack in Cuba," remarking that "researchers found that all of those reporting symptoms had evidence of cognitive dysfunction and an inner-ear abnormality" [28]. *USA Today* published the headline: "US Staff in Cuba Suffered Ear Damage, Study Says," and quoted Hoffer as saying, "We do know for sure that it's an injury to the ear and that the brain is affected," and went so far as to claim, "The evidence suggests that they were targeted" [29]. A military veteran with a security clearance,

Hoffer said he reached this conclusion "because they were being followed and the other individuals in their household were in some cases not affected" [30]. His co-author, Dr. Carey Balaban, a researcher in the department of Otolaryngology at the University of Pittsburgh, asserted that the study contained "measurable, quantifiable evidence that something really did happen. It's not just hysteria," he said [29].

Like the *JAMA* study published earlier in the year, these findings seemed to definitively resolve the question as to whether or not a nefarious attack took place in Cuba. The news media jumped on the story, reporting on what appeared to be a big break in the case of the American Embassy 'mystery illness,' but it too contained flaws – serious flaws. All 25 sufferers underwent a battery of tests focusing on their auditory and vestibular systems. While prior to the study's release, information was leaked to the press that nearly a third of the subjects had reported hearing loss as a result of their exposure to the events in Cuba, when the study was released, results of a standard hearing test found hearing loss in just two subjects. This finding is not surprising for any random group of 25 patients. What's more, both had hearing problems *before* the events in Cuba [25, p 5]. This discrepancy between what was leaked and what was found on the hearing test came about because many of the subjects under study believed they had suffered hearing loss from exposure to the mysterious sounds, when in reality, they had not. The authors provided no details on the subject's prior hearing loss or age. On the vestibular testing of balance and eye movement, they reported an array of ambiguous anomalies which, without an appropriate control group, are impossible to interpret and are essentially meaning-less. In other words, there was no baseline for comparison. As for the 10 housemates who did not report symptoms, inexplicably, they were not tested. Harvard Psychiatrist Dr. Janina Galler has expressed concern with the secrecy surrounding the study, which resulted in raw data not being shared with other scientists. "We don't have access even to the full sample size and how individuals were selected and why so many were not included in the study," she said [31]. With the exception of dizziness, which is notoriously difficult to measure, there was little overlap in the symptoms, suggestive of different causes instead of being targeted by some type of mysterious device.

When Dr. Hoffer's study was released, some Embassy staff who had been evacu-ated stateside, were upset by his statements and took exception with his claim that at the time he examined the Havana Embassy employees, their symptoms could not have been distorted or exaggerated because it had not been reported in the media and therefore they were "pure" and had not been contaminated from any ideas about what the potential symptoms could include. One staffer said: "This is false. The Embassy was a tightly-knit community with a very active rumor mill; many people were buzzing about the 'incidents' and the related ailments starting as far back as December 2016. We knew as far back as March or April…that doctors were com-paring the symptoms to Traumatic Brain Injury. We were absolutely primed to know what the symptoms were" [10].

Immediately after publication of the Hoffer-led study, a State Department spokesperson told the *Miami Herald* that the study had to be cleared by them to ensure that no sensitive classified information was revealed. However, there was an interesting twist: she said that the Department "was not requested to review nor did it receive a preliminary copy of the University of Miami's recent article regarding 'health attacks' for *Laryngoscope Investigative Otolaryngology*." It did, however, receive a similar article by Dr. Hoffer for clearance in December 2017, that was intended for submission to the *New England Journal of Medicine*. While the article was cleared on February 20, 2018, it was never published [32]. Despite the fact that *Laryngoscope Investigative Otolaryngology* had been published online for 3 years at the time the Hoffer-led study was published, it had yet to receive an impact ranking – the measure of how often its articles are cited in other publications in any given year. By any standard, it would be considered a low-impact journal. A perusal of their website also reveals that Hoffer sits on the editorial board. While none of these facts invalidates Hoffer's findings, it would appear that the study was rejected by the more prestigious *New England Journal of Medicine*, and then published in a journal with a less rigorous standard that is open to accepting pieces of a more speculate nature. When the study appeared, the London *Daily Mail* carried the headline: "It was NOT just Hysteria: Doctors Claim Cuba Sonic Attack Victims WERE Exposed to Something that Damaged their Ears and Brains - but the Cause Remains a Mystery." The paper's health editor, Mia de Graff lauded the findings, suggesting that it was somehow neutral and above the politics and controversy that was swirling around the issue, writing: "Their exams were done very early on, before any speculation about the cause had arisen, and before any prospective diagnoses had been given" [33]. Not only was speculation rampant among Embassy staff at the time of the study, but the interpretation of the findings and the way they conducted their retrospective review did not follow standard scientific protocols.

On September 7, 2018, prior to publication, Dr. Hoffer and Dr. Balaban discussed the findings and implications of their soon to be published article as part of a study program sponsored by the Pentagon. The ominous title of the program was: "Probable Use of a Neuroweapon to Affect Personnel of US Embassy in Havana: Findings, Pathology, Possible Causes and Disruptive Effects" [34]. According to Yahoo News, Pentagon officials stated that "the briefing was offered by the scientific team for interested people in the Defense Department and was to gain 'general knowledge' about their findings" [35]. After summarizing the clinical findings from the article, Hoffer noted: "It's important to know that the site of injury could be limited to the inner ear." He added, "the definition of mild traumatic brain injury as defined by the military does not fit these individuals" [35]. Hoffer concluded that their studies suggested damage to the gravity-sensing otolith organs of the inner ear which could explain the symptoms of dizziness and imbalance. But what could damage these otolith organs without affecting hearing and what is the evidence that selective otolith damage can cause dizziness? Neither the University of Pennsylvania nor the University of Miami teams could find evidence of hearing loss from the presumed "sonic attacks." Dr. Balaban suggested that some type of "directed energy weapon" could cause "air bubbles" in the inner ear [35]. But how would bubbles damage the relatively rigid otolith organ while sparing the delicate cochlea? Furthermore, there is no known clinical syndrome with selective damage to the otolith organs or with "bubbles" in the inner ear. It has been suggested that an ultrasonic device might be able to create 'acoustic bubbles' in the inner ear or even in the brain, causing damage. The world's leading expert on acoustic bubbles, Dr. Timothy Leighton, views such claims as science fiction. "If you put an ultrasound transducer next to a liquid, the way we do in ultrasonic cleaning baths, you can cause bubbles to form. But if you send it through the air, you will never get that effect. Acoustic bubbles only happen if you have direct contact. If someone goes for a pregnancy ultrasound, the doctor holds the transducer up against the body. They even have to put a slippery gel on the woman's abdomen, because if there is even a microscopic air gap, the ultrasound won't propagate" [36, p 44].

As to the type of directed energy weapon, the possibility of ultrasound, micro-waves, weaponized microbes, and drugs were all considered possible. Balaban suggested that commercial off-the-counter devices that could be picked up in your local department store such as insect repellent devices might do the trick. Another participant in the telephone conference, James Giordano, a professor of neurology and biochemistry at Georgetown University added "Is it possible and probable that ultrasonics can do this? Yes, it's very possible, and it's probable. Is it possible and probable that electromagnetic pulse devices that would then be propagated either directly or vectored could do this? Yes, it's very, very possible and very probable." The attacker could even customize the device to a specific person's head. "Could something like this be developed that actually models specific features that could then be precision or personalized? The answer to that question would be yes," Giordano said. "If you had anthropometric dimensions on a certain individual, that could be extracted, for example, from pictures" [36, p 44]. Some people have argued that the mysterious energy waves that are believed to have caused the illnesses in Cuba, were the result of The Frey Effect, named after Allan Frey, an American scientist who discovered that if microwaves are aimed at the human head, it can result in an audible clicking sound. Dr. Kenneth Foster, a Bioengineering Professor at the University of Pennsylvania has studied the effect and views claims that it could be involved in the Havana affair, as science fiction, noting that the sound would be barely audible. He told journalist Dan Hurley: "It is just a totally incredible explanation for what happened to these diplomats…It's just not possible. The idea that someone could beam huge amounts of microwave energy at people and not have it be obvious defies credibility. There's nothing behind it. You might as well say little green men from Mars were throwing darts of energy" [36, p 44]. The former head of the Electromagnetics division the Environmental Protection Agency, Ric Tell, has spent decades working on devising a set of international standards for safe exposure to electromagnetic radiation, including microwaves. He views the microwave claims with incredulity. "If a guy is standing in front of a high-powered radio antenna – and it's got to be high, really high — then he could experience his body getting warmer," Tell said. "But to cause brain-tissue damage, you would have to impart enough energy to heat it up to the point where it's cooking. I don't know how you could do that, especially if you were trying to transmit through a wall. It's just not plausible," he said [36, p 44].

In summary, the Cuban Embassy staff and their family members were examined by two different groups of doctors, ear specialists in Miami and brain trauma specialists in Philadelphia. The Miami team concluded that their symptoms were due to inner ear vestibular damage, and the Pennsylvania group attributed their symptoms to traumatic brain injury. Both groups claimed to have test results confirming their conclusions but on reviewing these results, the findings are vague, and they did not study appropriate control subjects. The one test that is reliable and reproducible and was performed by both groups, the audiogram or hearing test, was essentially normal, and any hearing loss was present before exposure. The idea that a "sonic attack" could cause inner ear vestibular damage or brain damage without affecting hearing is illogical. What the situation called for was a careful epidemiological study documenting exposure, that is, an examination of the incidence, frequency, and distribution of the symptoms and their causes, so a correlation could be made with each person's symptoms including an appropriate control group.

Aside from the shortcomings of the Swanson and Hoffer-led studies in *JAMA* and *Laryngoscope Investigative Otolaryngology* respectively, there were a number of behind-the-scenes issues between the two research teams. These issues should be acknowledged because some of the data they were basing their conclusions on was withheld on the grounds that the US government considered it to be potentially sensitive information. As a result, we are being asked to trust the researchers who had seen the data, and therefore their character and judgement can be considered a legitimate area of scrutiny. According to emails obtained by journalist Dan Vergano,"the teams quarrelled, refused to share data, and disagreed over study authorship, as they raced to publish in high-prestige publications" [37]. In the end, the team led by Swanson won the race, publishing on February 15, 2018, in the high profile *Journal of the American Medical Association*, while the Hoffer-led study had to settle for a December publication in an obscure journal after failing to be accepted by the *New England Journal of Medicine*. One issue of contention between the two teams involved authorship and prompted Dr. Carey Balaban and fellow team members Michael Hoffer and Bonnie Levin at the University of Miami, to pull the plug on their association with the *JAMA* study.

In January 2018, Hoffer, Balaban, and Levin received notification from the journal editors that an article had been submitted by the Penn team and that they were listed as co-authors. They needed them to sign off on the necessary forms such as attestation of authorship, to insure they were included. This prompted a series of heated exchanges between Balaban and Smith over the appropriateness of such a move. A week before the study was published online, Dr. Douglas Smith wrote to Balaban telling him that he, Hoffer and Levin needed to make up their minds quickly on whether to be included. The header in the e-mail was blunt: "in or out." Balaban wrote back to express concern that he was being listed as an author of the study, yet his repeated requests to see the data it was based on, were denied, raising questions surrounding "ethical standards for research and academic integrity to authorship rights and responsibilities." Balaban pleaded with Smith to understand his predicament: "Please understand the ethical dilemma that you have presented to me. The acknowledgements state that I shared responsibility for 'Acquisition, analysis, or interpretation of data' and 'Critical revision of the manuscript for important intellectual content.' However, my repeated requests to see the data, initiated when I first saw the manuscript in mid-January, have been ignored and you have expressed an unwillingness to entertain any interpretative input or suggestions for revision" [38]. Balaban wanted Smith to delay publication and to see the data. He then raised the spectre of an investigation into scientific misconduct, writing that he was sharing their correspondence with ethics officials at Balaban's home institution the University of Pittsburgh. Smith fired back that they were lucky to be offered inclusion, noting that "you did not participate in acquisition or analysis of any of the data that appears in the manuscript. Indeed, if you were to be an author, we had a completely different justification for your efforts based only on legacy efforts" from early involvement. Smith then made it clear that while he was willing to allow their authorship, they were fortunate to even get that. "Authorship on the paper for you is essentially a gift, yet you continue to search for some leverage where you have none" [39].

In the end, Balaban, Hoffer, and Levin opted out and their names were removed from the *JAMA* study [37], and Balaban filed a complaint with University of Pittsburgh ethics officials [40]. On the day the study appeared online, Balaban complained to a colleague about potential unethical practices, writing: "An interesting story behind the headlines. To my surprise, I was listed as an author on the original submission without ever having seen the paper. When I inquired further, I was repeatedly denied the opportunity to look at data or suggest revisions to the manuscript. Rather, I was told that authorship was being offered as a 'gift.' Hence, I could not ethically sign the attestation of authorship requested by the journal (i.e., accept a 'gift' to commit academic misconduct). A repeated refusal to show data to a designated 'co-author' is troubling, per se. As we both know, there can be many 'devils in the details' of data interpretation of a novel and perplexing phenomenon" [41].

Another area of controversy and potential conflict of interest centers around diagnostic goggles that were developed by Hoffer and Balaban in conjunction with Neuro Kinetics, a Pittsburgh-based company that develops diagnostic and assessment tools for neurologists. The goggles were being developed prior to the outbreak of illness in Cuba and were being advertised on the Neuro Kinetics website in 2015 as "Concussion-Goggles" that were "Game-Changing Technology" that could assist in the rapid assessment of concussion, whether it was on the playing field or the battlefield [42]. On November 5, 2015, CBS-TV in Miami did a feature story on the goggles [43]. FDA approval was granted in November 2017. The experimental goggles were used by Hoffer in his 2018 study of embassy patients and were clearly a potential conflict of interest that should have been declared. It is not clear what Balaban and Hoffer stood to gain from the device. In one test, the goggles project moving points of light while a camera assesses eye movement. While healthy subjects are able to track the lights, those with concussion often find it difficult to focus on them [24]. Cuban neurologist Mitchell Valdés-Sosa sees the goggles as relevant to 'Havana Syndrome.' "There could be a conflict of interest, and that could have [led] to confirmation bias," where researchers see what they expect to see in their patients. "Their hypothesis could have been that they were going to find evidence of vestibular [inner ear] damage, which is what the [Neuro Kinetics] helmet measures." Even if there was not a vested interest financially, given their role in helping to develop them, there must have been an emotional interest [37].

Ear-Witness Testimony

The implications of the Golden study are significant given the ambiguous nature of the sounds that were experienced by the first few diplomats – sounds that would later be assumed to have been the result of sonic harassment either by or with the knowledge of the Cuban government. Human visual and auditory perception are notoriously unreliable and subject to error. It is well known within the field of social psychology and criminology that visual perception is fallible: thousands of people have been wrongly convicted based on eye-witness testimony, only to have DNA evidence exonerate them. In some cases, the wrongly accused had already been executed. While less known, a similar situation exists with ear-witness testimony. It too is unreliable to the extent that in some studies, people were unable to even correctly identify the voices of family members [44]. In discussing the results of a series of studies on the accuracy of audio information, Lisa Öhman of the Department of Psychology at the University of Gothenburg in Sweden found that "after testing a total of 949 witnesses under a number of different conditions, the message is clear; voice identification under reasonably realistic conditions is a highly difficult task. Actors in the legal system should, therefore, treat voice identification evidence with caution" [45]. The variation in the sounds that were reported by the diplomats, were very diverse and included such descriptions as buzzing, grinding and a high-pitched whine. However, many of the recordings by those who claimed to have taped the 'attacks,' were suspiciously similar to the sounds made by crickets and cicadas. Insects and sounds have a long history of triggering episodes of mass psychogenic illness and social panics as we will discuss in Chaps. 6, 7 and 9. Just as the nocebo effect has the power to make people feel sick when they have no underlying physical ailment, the human mind has the propensity to hear and see things that do not exist.

The Context: Ghosts of the Cold War Past

During the Cold War, there were many attempts by US agents to destabilize the regime of Cuban President Fidel Castro including the failed CIA-backed Bay of Pigs invasion in 1961 and several unsuccessful assassination attempts that included a poison cigar, and an exploding seashell (Castro loved to scuba-dive and was to be lured to the shell) [46]. Cuban agents responded with a series of ongoing actions that are well-known in the diplomatic corps. As a result, despite reopening the American Embassy in Havana under the Obama Administration on July 20, 2015, and the promise of a new era in relations that it was to usher in, diplomats stationed in Havana were aware that they were working in a foreign country that had a long history of antagonizing US Embassy staff. The Embassy in Havana was closed in 1961 when President Dwight Eisenhower cut ties with the Castro government after his rise to power. During this period, the US managed to maintain a diplomatic presence on the island in the form of a mission at the United States Interests Section in Havana. The actions of Cuban agents against embassy personnel have been well-documented to the point where it has become part of American Intelligence folklore. Diplomats were harassed in a myriad of ways. Cuban agents were known to enter their homes, rearrange books and furniture, dump urine or feces onto the floor, deflate car tires, and find ways to disrupt their sleep. Sometimes they would turn off your electricity or water. On other occasions, they would tailgate your car or shine lights into your motor vehicle or home at night [47–49]. CIA operative Jason Matthews who once served in Havana, recalls how he would wake up in the morning and walk into the living room, only to find cigarette butts on his coffee table ashtray – an intentional message left by Cuban agents tasked with watching his every move [50]. One Embassy staffer in Cuba told us that once news of the 'attacks' got out, "many of us *were* experiencing headaches, mental fog, irritability, etc.," and this was "completely understandable given the high stress environment and the fact that we went asleep every night wondering whether we'd be zapped in our beds, and consequently lay awake for hours at a time, days on end, stretching into weeks and months" [10]. One employee told of feeling extreme guilt for having brought their child with them and wondering whether or not their health would be impacted as a result. They described the situation as terrifying [10]. In a 2007 report, the State Department's Inspector General wrote that "life in Havana is life with a government that 'lets you know it's hostile." It mentioned other acts of harassment ranging "from the petty to the poisoning of family pets." The report also made an important observation: "All employees are fully aware that host government hostility extends to an elaborate, aggressive intelligence apparatus" [49]. The head of the US Interests Section in the years prior to the 2015 thaw in relations, John Caulfield, said that American diplomats in Cuba know that while they are on assignment there, they are under 24-hour surveillance [49]. One declassified US government cable read: "In one example that demonstrates how regime officials actually listen to the daily activities of the [U.S. diplomatic] staff, presumably through electronic bugs, shortly after one family discussed the susceptibility of their daughter to mosquito bites, they returned home to find all of their windows open and the house full of mosquitoes" [51].

US Embassy staff in Cuba were a close-knit group sharing a common work environment in an atmosphere of high stress in a foreign country where they knew they were being constantly watched. As one former diplomat who served in the American Embassy in Havana observed: "Cuba is considered a high-threat, high-stress post… Before we go to Cuba, it is drilled into our heads: There will be surveillance. There will be listening devices in your house, probably in your car. Assume they are always watching. For some people, that puts them in a high-stress mentality, in a threat-anticipation mode" [52]. Cuba is also a country with a recent and lengthy history of hostile actions against Americans working there, so when staff members initially became aware of the threat, it would have seemed plausible, and the natural assumption was that it must have been the Cubans up to their old tricks again. The counseling of future Embassy staff over the perceived threat created an expectation of illness, and with it, a new frame through which future sounds and symptoms were interpreted. As is typical in mass psychogenic illness outbreaks, as news of the 'attacks' spread among the diplomatic community, more US Embassy staff were affected. Many 'incidents' were said to have occurred in homes and hotels. Why were some people affected, while others either standing or sleeping next to the 'victim,' were not? This irregular patterning is not characteristic of an infectious agent. Even more conspicuous is why non-diplomats at either the American or Canadian embassies were not affected.

One of the major factors in assuming that a sonic attack took place was what State Department officials viewed as a series of unusual events that were deemed unlikely to have been coincidence: the first few Americans who were affected were working with the CIA in a small station in Havana. Based on interviews with US government officials, he observes: "The suspicious fact that CIA officers seemed to have been struck first and disproportionately by the strange sounds and illnesses – at least four people connected to the small Havana station reported symptoms, as well as a CIA employee who came to the island on temporary duty later on – led agency officials to assume that the incidents were some kind of harassment or electronic-monitoring effort directed at intelligence officers" [52]. State Department officials failed to realize that this pattern is a defining feature of mass psychogenic illness, which is known to follow social networks. Outbreaks commonly begin in small social groups and spread outward, starting with people of higher status. All the telltale signs of psychogenic illness were there, but they had not put the pieces together. Instead of searching for mundane causes, they focused on exotic explanations.

From Sonic Attacks to Microwaves

In Early September 2018, one of the authors of the *JAMA* study, Dr. Douglas Smith, suddenly latched onto the microwave explanation. On September 1, the *New York Times* carried the headline: "Microwave Weapons are Prime Suspect in Ills of US Embassy Workers." Smith told the *Times* that microwave radiation could be the culprit. There was only one problem with his interview: he provided no supporting evidence. According to Kenneth Foster, Professor of Bioengineering at the University of Pennsylvania, the microwave explanation is "a real stretch" as it would require "a major airport radar transmitter with the subject's head close to the antenna in its direct beam" [53]. While technically possible, it is highly improbable. Those reporting symptoms were not even at the Embassy, but in their own homes or in one of two major Havana hotels. The microwave explanation was so unconvincing that it was never even considered in the *JAMA* study by Dr. Smith and his colleagues.

If one scours the internet, they will find many claims about the American military engaging in secret experiments with microwave weapons. The science journal *Nature* has published a review on the progress of the development of microwave weapons. It concluded that "Despite 50 years of research on high-powered microwaves, the US military has yet to produce a usable weapon," and referred to it as "Wasted Energy" [54]. The author of the review, Sharon Weinberger, is the Washington Bureau Chief for Yahoo News. She is an expert on the history of the US military's development of microwave weapons [55]. She reports that the situation remains the same today. After the publication of the *New York Times* article speculating on a possible link between microwaves and the sick diplomats, Weinberger Tweeted that "American work on U.S. microwave weapons intended to target humans has been an unmitigated disaster... Filled with secrecy, overblown claims, and ultimately weapons of questionable utility, like the Active Denial System, which was never deployed on the battlefield" [56]. Even if such a weapon existed, it would be impossible to target individuals deep inside one of the two large hotels in Havana, as has been claimed.

References

1. Richardson DJ. The complete midsummer night's dream: an annotated edition of the Shakespeare play. Bloomington: Authorhouse; 2013. p. 155.
2. Attacks on U.S. diplomats in Cuba: response and oversight. US Senate Committee on Foreign Relations, Subcommittee on Western Hemisphere, Transnational Crime, Civilian Security, Democracy, Human Rights, and Global Women's Issues. Attacks on US diplomats in Cuba. Video of the complete hearing published 2018 Jan 9. https://www.c-span.org/video/?439474-1/state-department-officials-testify-attacks-us-diplomats-cuba. Accessed 22 Oct 2019.
3. Weissenstein M. US senator says 'no evidence' of sonic attacks in Cuba. The Washington Post. 6 Jan 2018.
4. Oppmann P, Koran L. Senate holds hearing on Cuba 'sonic attacks. CNN. 9 Jan 2018.
5. Official Twitter feed of Marco Rubio. https://twitter.com/marcorubio?lang=en. 7 Jan 2018.
6. Dorsey S. Pentagon turns focus to Cuba health 'attacks' amid new findings on American victims. CBS News. 2018 Sept 12. https://www.cbsnews.com/news/pentagon-turns-focus-to-cuba-attacks/. Accessed 22 Oct 2019.
7. Moore WW. Wise sayings: for your thoughtful consideration. Bloomington: Authorhouse; 2011. p. 1–2.
8. Lippmann W. Public opinion. Mineola: Dover; 2004. p. 7.
9. Oppmann P, Labott E. US diplomats, families in Cuba targeted nearly 50 times by sonic attacks, says US official. CNN News. 23 Sept 2017.
10. Interview between Robert Bartholomew and a U.S. Embassy employee who was stationed in Havana during the 'attacks' and wishes to remain anonymous.
11. Swanson R, Hampton S, Green-McKenzie J, Diaz-Arrastia R, Grady M, Ragini V, et al. Neurological manifestations among US government personnel reporting directional audible and sensory phenomena in Havana, Cuba. JAMA. 2018;319(11):1125–33. https://doi.org/10.1001/jama.2018.1742.
12. Fields RD. Sonic weapon attacks on U.S. embassy don't add up – for anyone. Sci Am. 16 Feb 2018.
13. Muth C, Lewis SL. Editorial: neurological symptoms among US diplomats in Cuba. JAMA. 2018;319(11):1098–100. https://doi.org/10.1001/jama.2018.1780.
14. Della Sala S, Cubelli R. Alleged 'sonic attack' supported by poor neuropsychology. Cortex. 2018;103:387–8. https://doi.org/10.1016/j.cortex.2018.03.006.
15. Hiltzik M. Is junk science adding to the mystery of the Havana embassy attacks? The Los Angeles Times. 12 June 2018.
16. Rubin R. More questions raised by concussion-like symptoms found in US diplomats who served in Havana. JAMA. 2018;319(11):1079.
17. Reed G. What happened to the US diplomats in Havana? Mitchell Valdés MD PhD Director, Cuban Neuroscience Center. Int J Cuban Health Med. 2018;20(4):14–9.
18. Sample I. What happened to US diplomats in Cuba? The Guardian. Science weekly podcast. 2018 Feb 23. https://www.theguardian.com/science/audio/2018/feb/23/what-happened-to-us-diplomats-in-cuba-science-weekly-podcast. Accessed 21 Sept 2019.

19. Cortex Editorial Board. Responsibility of neuropsychologists: the case of the 'sonic attack'. Cortex. 2018;108:A1–2. https://doi.org/10.1016/j.cortex.2018.10.001.
20. The statement in the JAMA rebuttal, which was considered confusing, ambiguous, and problematic, was as follows: *"Within-individual deviations from an average performance are considered signs of brain dysfunction. Percentile scores in our report showed that all impaired patients had several scores that deviated by more than 1 SD from their respective means, some exceeding 2 SDs, which translates to more than 40 percentile points below their means (below 10th percentile relative to their average performance). This meets standard criteria for neuropsychological impairment ..."* (from Hampton S, Swanson R, Smith DH. In reply. JAMA. 2018;320(6):604–5.
21. Della Sala S, McIntosh RD, Cubelli R, Kacmarski JA, Miskey HM, Shura RD. Cognitive symptoms in US government personnel in Cuba: the mending is worse than the hole. Cortex. 2018;108:287–8. https://doi.org/10.1016/j.cortex.2018.10.002.
22. Golden T, Rotella S. The sound and the fury: inside the mystery of the Havana embassy. ProPublica. 2018 Feb 14. https://www.propublica.org/article/diplomats-in-cuba. Accessed 11 Nov 2019.
23. Hitt J. Hear no evil. Vanity Fair. 2019 Feb;61(2):48. https://www.vanityfair.com/news/2019/01/the-real-story-behind-the-havana-embassy-mystery. Accessed 22 Oct 2019.
24. Stone R. Sonic attack or mass paranoia? Science. 2018. https://doi.org/10.1126/science.aau5386.
25. Hoffer ME, Levin BE, Snapp H, Buskirk J, Balaban C. Acute findings in an acquired neurosensory dysfunction. Laryngoscope Investig Otolaryngol. 2018;1–8 (12 Dec).
26. Burke P. Physicians announce clinical findings of 'sonic' attacks at US embassy in Cuba. WPLG Channel 10 News, Pembroke (FL). 12 Dec 2018.
27. University of Miami medical team reports acute findings from the Havana embassy phenomenon. Press release, University of Miami, Miller School of Medicine. 12 Dec 2018.
28. Lardieri A. U.S. diplomats show inner-ear damage after mysterious sonic attack in Cuba. U.S. News & World Report. 12 Dec 2018.
29. Stanglin D. US staff in Cuba suffered ear damage. USA Today. 14 Dec 2018;Sect. A3.
30. Robles F. U.S. diplomats with mysterious illness in Cuba had inner-ear damage, doctors say. The New York Times. 13 Dec 2018.
31. Hamilton J. Doubts about evidence that U.S. diplomats in Cuba were attacked. All Things Considered. National public radio program airing on March 25, 2019. https://www.npr.org/sections/health-shots/2019/03/25/704903613/doubts-rise-about-evidence-that-u-s-diplomats-in-cuba-were-attacked. Accessed 5 Apr 2019.
32. Gámez Torres N. Doctors who first tested diplomats after Cuba 'health attacks' doubt concussion theory. Miami Herald. 12 Dec 2018.
33. de Graff M. It was not just hysteria: doctors claim Cuba sonic attack victims were exposed to something that damaged their ears and brains - but the cause remains a mystery. The Daily Mail (London). 13 Dec 2018.
34. Balaban C. Probable use of a neuroweapon to affect personnel of US embassy in Havana: findings, pathology, possible causes and disruptive effects. Teleconference, Strategic Multi-Layer Assessment for the United States Joint Chiefs of Staff and Department of Defense. 7 Sept 2018.
35. Weinberger S. Scientists say 'neuroweapons' were behind Cuba attacks. Yahoo News. 10 Sept 2018.
36. Hurley D. The diplomat's disorder. The New York Times Magazine. 19 May 2019, p. 40–5, 71.
37. Vergano D. The US government botched its investigation into the mysterious 'sonic attack' in Cuba, emails reveal. BuzzFeed News. 29 May 2019. We are grateful to Mr. Vergano for sharing some of these emails.
38. Re: in or out. Email from Carey Balaban to Douglas Smith. 9 Feb 2018.
39. Re: in or out. Email from Douglas Smith to Carey Balaban. 9 Feb 2018.
40. The ethics investigation was confirmed to Dan Vergano by Joe Miksch, Director of Media Relations at the University of Pittsburgh. Personal communication with Dan Vergano. 1 Nov 2019.

41. Breaking: medical findings in U.S. government personnel... E-mail from Carey Balaban to Kurt Yankaskas. 16 Feb 2018.
42. See the following advertisement for the goggles. 2015 Nov 26. https://neuro-kinetics.com/project/game-changing-technology-concussion-goggles/. Accessed 30 Oct 2019.
43. Cugno M. Game-changing technology: concussion goggles. Miami (FL): CBS4 News TV. 5 Nov 2015.
44. McClelland E. Voice recognition within a closed set of family members. Paper presented at the International Association for Forensic phonetics and Acoustics (IAFPA) Conference, Swiss Federal Institute of Technology Lausanne. Lausanne, Switzerland, July 2008.
45. Öhman L. All ears: adults' and children's earwitness testimony. Sweden: Department of Psychology, University of Gothenburg; 2013, piii.
46. Campbell D. Close but no cigar: how America failed to kill Fidel Castro. The Guardian 26 Nov 2016.
47. Robles F, Semple K. 'Health attacks' on U.S. diplomats in Cuba baffle both countries. The New York Times. 11 Aug 2017.
48. Bruno J. The foreign circus. Canastota: Bittersweet House Press; 2004.
49. Weissenstein W, Lee M. Tillerson says diplomats in Havana suffered 'health attacks.' The Associated Press News. 12 Aug 2017.
50. Entous A. Exploding mojitos: the first 'sonic attacks' targeting American diplomats in Cuba may have taken place thirty years ago. The New Yorker. 12 Nov 2018.
51. Rosenberg C. U.S. details harassment of diplomats in Cuba. Miami Herald. 6 Feb 2003.
52. Golden T, Rotella S. The strange case of American diplomats in Cuba: as the mystery deepens, so do divisions in Washington. 9 Nov 2018.
53. Mosbergen D. Microwave weapons could be the culprit behind the mysterious U.S. embassy attacks. The Huffington Post. 2 Sept 2018.
54. Weinberger S. Wasted energy. Nature. 2012;489:198–200. (13 Sept)
55. Weinberger S. The imagineers of war: the untold story of DARPA, the pentagon agency that changed the world. New York: Vintage; 2018.
56. Weinberger S. Tweet dated 2018 Sept 2 from @weinbergersa.

Canadian Contagion

3

Talk of the devil and he is bound to appear.

–English proverb

In April 2017, Canadian embassy staff and their families began developing symptoms similar to the Americans, after a Canadian embassy employee was informally alerted about the attacks by his American neighbor and the employee passed the information on to his embassy. Although rumors had been circulating in Havana about strange attacks on the Americans, the Canadians had not been concerned since they were on friendly terms with the Cuban government. An email to Ottawa in mid-May, approved by the Canadian ambassador, suggested that some Canadians may have been experiencing psychosomatic symptoms. It read in part: "Many of the symptoms are similar to signs of extreme stress, and there is the possibility that there could be mental health effects caused by the fear of being targeted. Either way, testing should help to rule out cases and reassure personnel that we have the means to be able to provide duty of care" [1]. But when others began developing mysterious symptoms, they became alarmed. A diplomat who spoke to the *Toronto Star* on the condition of anonymity said, "The stress has been awful. We feel we have been abandoned. I expect my government to be concerned about my well-being" [2]. The *Star* reported that the Canadian family that had been warned by their American neighbors in April, themselves became the target in June. "After the Americans left, the Canadian family had suffered a frightening night-time 'attack' that left some in the house feeling nauseated and suffering nosebleeds" [2]. Affected family members were flown to Miami "where testing revealed they had suffered brain injuries" [2]. After this incident, Canadian embassy staff were called together and told to be on the lookout for strange noises and if they heard anything, to move to other parts of the house and not to go outside to investigate. Any unusual symptoms should be reported to senior officials. However, embassy staff complained that no precautions were being taken and they suspected that the embassy was trying to downplay the whole problem. But people were becoming sick with a range of symptoms. "You felt crappy. It wasn't like a headache. It was waves of pain that came and went

© Springer Nature Switzerland AG 2020
R. W. Baloh, R. E. Bartholomew, *Havana Syndrome*,
https://doi.org/10.1007/978-3-030-40746-9_3

throughout the day," said one affected staff member [2]. Frustrated with the Canadian response, two staffers paid their own airfare to the University of Pennsylvania brain trauma center for evaluation. Their tests showed "the same concussion-like effects as the Americans, including neurological, balance, vestibular and other problems." [2] In April 2018, Canadian diplomatic staff in Havana were no longer allowed to have their families accompany them while posted in Havana. The *Toronto Star* alarmingly described the situation as "a mysterious series of attacks seemingly taken from the pages of a Cold War spy thriller" [3].

The Canadian's homes were located all over the city, so any weapon would have to have been moved around without anyone noticing. Dr. Smith, director of the University of Pennsylvania Department of Neurosurgery and Center for Brain Injury and Repair was a senior author of the *JAMA* study and told the *Star* since there was no likely environmental cause, he suspected "something nefarious" [3]. He admitted that initially he and his colleagues were skeptical, but they became convinced that the symptoms were "real" and impossible to fake. They were "indistinguishable" from symptoms in patients treated in their concussion clinic. "People started calling this immaculate concussion," Smith said. He was particularly impressed with the "directional aspect" of the attacks and that the sensation would disappear if the person moved to another room or behind a concrete wall. "Toxins and infections don't do that. It supports the idea of a directed energy type of exposure," he said [3]. Although many Canadians also reported hearing noises at the onset of their symptoms, Smith didn't think that the noise was the culprit. "Audible sound cannot hurt your brain," he said. "It happened at the same time as another type of exposure that did injure the brain" [3]. But what other type of exposure could cause brain injury? Canadian and American diplomatic quarters in Havana were investigated for environmental toxins including air and water samples and the Royal Canadian Mounted Police and the FBI performed detailed searches for a sound source or any other device that might injure the brain. Nothing was found.

In late January 2019, the Canadian Government announced that a fourteenth member of their diplomatic staff in Havana had been "confirmed" to have mysterious health complaints paralleling those that had sickened the American Embassy workers there, and later in China. In response, Canada cut its Havana mission staff from 16 to 8. Within a week, lawyers acting on behalf of the 14–5 diplomats and their families, had filed a $28 million lawsuit (US$21 million) [4–6]. The suit claimed that the Canadian government knew of the risks in early 2017, and had failed to protect their citizens in the face of the clear and present danger of "Havana Syndrome." It was asserted that the victims had been targeted in their homes and were suffering from the same array of symptoms as were the Americans who had been evacuated. This included "traumatic brain injuries." The suit read: "Throughout the crisis, Canada downplayed the seriousness of the situation, hoarded and concealed critical health and safety information, and gave false, misleading and incomplete information to diplomatic staff" [7, p 4]. It went on to criticize claims that they were the victims of mass suggestion, contending that Canadian officials deliberately suggested that they had been victimized by their own imaginations, causing them pain and injuring their reputations [7, p 4].

As with the American staffers, the Canadians reported a vast assortment of symptoms, most of which are common in the general population. For instance, a female diplomat and her son were described as suffering from "Havana Syndrome," yet their complaints were remarkably vague and common. The woman said that she "began regularly experiencing strange sensations in her ear lasting seconds, followed by waves of uncomfortable pressure in her ear that would last for minutes." These would often happen in the evening and during the middle of the night. She also experienced nausea, dizziness, ringing in the ears, pain behind the eyes, difficulty speaking, exhaustion, memory problems and issues with her vision. She said that during the 'attacks,' her son felt "waves of pressure," prompting him to "cover his ears and groan" [7, p 18]. The symptoms that the group of 14 were said to have experienced included neurological complaints resembling brain injuries, headaches and migraines, dizziness, balance problems, nausea, insomnia, fatigue, difficulty remembering and concentrating, emotional disturbances including depression, irritability, anger, anxiety, sadness, nervousness, worry, ear pain, tinnitus, sensitivity to light and sound, vision problems, nose bleeds, and even "loss of consciousness" [7, pp 21–22]. Most of these symptoms would be routinely encountered by a GP, yet this did not stop the lawyers from claiming that the plaintiffs were "clearly the victims of some kind of new weaponry, or method of attack" [7, p 21]. In any given week, many people in the general population would experience more than one of these symptoms. Athletes would often exhibit many of the same symptoms prior to and during sporting competitions, while students commonly experience similar complaints in preparing for and taking high school and university exams.

60 Minutes Enters the Fray

On Sunday, March 17, 2019, CBS aired a sensational segment of their news magazine *60 Minutes* on what it claimed was evidence that a hostile foreign government was targeting American diplomats in both Havana and China with a mysterious energy source [8]. Several diplomats who had been stationed in China told of falling ill after hearing mysterious sounds. The trouble is, they interviewed people with an array of complaints that are found in the general population including a man with Parkinson's disease, a toddler who had fallen twice in the same day ("She never does that," her mother said), a man with pre-existing head trauma, and a women who complained of dizziness and ear problems which coincided with the appearance of a skin rash. American Neuroscientist R. Douglas Fields of the National Institutes of Health was critical of the report and the exotic suggestion that they had been "targeted and injured by a clandestine energy beam weapon" [9]. The report also stated that "The FBI is now investigating whether these Americans were attacked by a mysterious weapon that leaves no trace." They left out that the FBI had revealed nearly a year earlier that they found no evidence to support claims that any type of attack had taken place in Cuba [10]. There were several references to the University of Pennsylvania study that was published in the *Journal of the American Medical Association* and their findings of "brain injury" in the Havana Embassy patients, but not a single criticism or even a hint that their conclusions were contentious.

The framing of the story drew the ire of Fields. During the previous month, he had attended the American Association for the Advancement of Science annual meeting which brought together American and Cuban scientists to discuss the evidence. While CBS News and *60 Minutes* were fully aware of the meeting and its conclusions, they left out that delegates found that the attack claims were *not* supported by the evidence. Fields was aghast by the one-sided nature of the *60 Minutes* report, considering it tantamount to journalistic malpractice. "On the basis of the current evidence, the panel roundly rejected the fear that these people have suffered brain injury from a mysterious energy beam weapon. …that *60 Minutes* had information from this meeting of scientists, but chose not to present it in their program, makes their report a lie of omission. That is a disservice to the public, to their profession, and to their once honorable reputation" [9, 11].

Segment producers Oriana Zill de Granados and Michael Rey said they had worked diligently on the report for over a year, compiling evidence of a hostile government attack against Embassy staff in both China and Cuba. In dismissing mass suggestion, they noted that young children and family pets had been affected. However, the symptoms were so varied and vague, it would be difficult for a child not to exhibit some of the complaints – whether they were aware of the attack claims or not. Nausea, headache, fatigue, trouble sleeping, and ear problems including pressure and pain are common childhood ailments. As for pets experiencing similar symptoms, given the ambiguity of many of the complaints, it is difficult to determine just how one's Cocker Spaniel is feeling on any given day. How does one know, for instance, that their dog is experiencing nausea or is suffering from a headache when they cannot speak? One of the diplomats in China dismissed the mass hysteria hypothesis by noting that her dog had vomited and could not have been influenced by media coverage about the symptoms, yet vomiting was not one of the complaints listed in Cuba. Zill de Granados said that she and Rey had "been incredibly careful to check everything we can," yet the segment treats the University of Pennsylvania study as Gospel. They failed to present a single skeptical voice from the many scientists who have been outspoken critics of the study and published critiques of it in a later edition of the very same journal [12]. These criticisms appeared 7 months before the *60 Minutes* segment aired and included concerns raised by the likes of British Neurologist Jon Stone and Neuropsychiatrist Alan Carson, German Neurologist Stoyan Popkirov, American Psychologist Robert Shura, and one of the authors (Bartholomew) [13–17].

Unsound Science: The Second *JAMA* Study

On July 23, 2019, JAMA published a second study of US Embassy diplomats who fell ill under mysterious circumstances while working in Cuba. A team of scientists including some who were involved in the original 2018 *JAMA* study, conducted sophisticated MRI scans on the brains of 40 diplomats who reported symptoms. *The real mystery of this study was how, after receiving a torrent of criticism* of their earlier publication, the editors could have approved such a flawed second study. Once again, their findings generated alarming international headlines as researchers found that their white matter volume had shrunk by about 5 percent, while their auditory networks exhibited a 15 percent reduction in function. The researchers wrote that "imaging revealed significant differences in whole brain white matter volume, regional gray and white matter volumes, cerebellar tissue microstructural integrity, and functional connectivity in the auditory and visuospatial subnetworks" *when compared to a group of healthy controls* [18, p 336]. To the layperson and journalists who were not neurologists or experts on brain function, this highly technical study could easily be seen as confirmation that something sinister had transpired in Cuba. Indeed, publication of the study prompted a flurry of media reports which gave credence to the acoustical attack claims. For instance, Britain's *Sun* newspaper reported that the mysterious 'sonic attacks' had left US embassy staff in Cuba "with shrunken brains" [19]. The *New York Post* proclaimed: "Cuba 'Sonic Attacks' Changed US Diplomats' Brains, Study Finds" [20]. *New Scientist* heralded: "Brain Scans Hint the Mysterious 'Sonic Attack' in Cuba was Real" [21]. Reuters quoted the study's lead author, Dr. Ragini Verma, as describing differences in the brains of the two groups as "jaw-dropping" [22]. However, this was not borne out by the data as differences between the two groups were relatively minor. This finding was buried in the limitations section where the researchers were forced to acknowledge that "…it cannot be determined whether the differences…are due to individual differences between patients or differences in level and degree of exposure to an uncharacterized directional phenomenon." In other words, the differences could be potentially explained by individual variation. Curiously, this limitation was never mentioned in the abstract, which gave the impression that affected embassy staff had brain abnormalities that could not be accounted for. At the very least, the wording made it appear as if there was more of a mystery than there was. The study was rife with methodological flaws and claims that were not supported by the evidence. While they found brain anomalies, their significance was unclear. Brain changes do not equate to brain damage, and 12 of those affected had pre-existing histories of concussion, compared to *none* of the healthy controls. This alone could account for the differences between the two groups. Furthermore, an array of conditions can generate similar neurological abnormalities when compared to healthy controls, many of them common – from migraines to chronic dizziness to depression. British Neurologist Jon Stone was incredulous of the findings, noting that such studies cannot determine if there was a brain injury [23, 24].

Another concern was the use of complex computer models to generate their findings – which was necessary as the patients were not given routine MRI scans. The researchers used advanced brain imaging that is notoriously difficult to interpret as it produces a massive number of data points that unlike regular MRIs, are so complex they can only be understood with sophisticated computer programs. False positives are as high as 70 percent and have prompted computer scientists to caution that many of these programs have critical design flaws [25]. Dr. Verma acknowledges that the 2018 *JAMA* scans of 21 embassy staff using conventional MRIs, were unrevealing, hence, the use of advanced imaging techniques that are usually only used in scientific research. Even if we disregard the reliance on these computer models, the healthy control group was not appropriate as performing these studies in *any* group of patients with symptoms caused by *any* illness would lead to comparable differences with healthy controls – and this includes psychogenic illness. The authors admit that the clinical relevance of their findings is unclear and the relationship to any exposure (auditory or otherwise) is unknown. Neurologist Sergio Della Sala was underwhelmed by the findings, noting that the differences between the two groups could be explained by differences in life experiences that can result in brain changes – including learning a foreign language [26]. As with the earlier *JAMA* study, the authors of the 2019 report refer to exposure to a "directional phenomena" as the cause of the symptoms even though they provide no information on what that could be. The researchers *assume* that embassy personnel were exposed to a mysterious energy source – a claim that is entirely without foundation. The abstract began by stating matter-of-factly that "United States government personnel experienced potential exposures to uncharacterized directional phenomena while serving in Havana" and that their study was intended to compare differences in those who had been exposed "with individuals not exposed to directional phenomena" [22, 27].

Despite these issues, several major media outlets carried dramatic stories on the study, giving the impression that Embassy staff had been exposed to some type of energy force that had left them with impaired brain function. The *Times* of London published the headline, "US Envoys in Cuba have Brain Damage." In the article, science editor Tom Whipple interviewed Dr. Douglas H. Smith, who was involved in both *JAMA* studies. He said the findings were vindication after the first study was criticized by experts, particularly those who pointed out the psychogenic features of the outbreak. "The patients feel they've been attacked twice. Many individuals who heard about the story, without examining the patients, made very strident claims it was all psychological," he said. On the other hand, "everyone in our group who examined the individuals feel it is a neurological disorder" [28]. After interviewing Dr. Randel Swanson, who also took part in both studies, journalist Peter Hess wrote that the findings had eliminated "mass hysteria" as a possible cause. Swanson stated that "The pattern is so consistent that it would be astronomically hard for all these individuals from various walks of life to systematically fool all these experts." Such statements are woefully ignorant of the literature on psychogenic illness and assume that the patients were feigning illness [29]. In Canada, the *Ottawa Citizen* carried the headline, "'Not Just in their Heads:' Scientists find Anomalies in Brains of 'Havana Syndrome' Patients" [30]. It cannot be over-emphasized that while there remains a stigma attached to psychogenic explanations and while such diagnoses may be unpopular, they are a perfectly legitimate medical condition. Just because someone exhibits psychogenic symptoms, does not mean they are not experiencing real symptoms, are mentally weak or are psychologically disturbed. Smith's statement shows a fundamental lack of understanding of functional disorders in general and mass psychogenic illness in specific. His views are a reflection of popular culture.

Dr. Smith also continued to assert that what was seen in the Embassy patients was unique in the annals of medicine. He told *The Daily Telegraph* that "These types of changes are completely unknown to us…We haven't seen anything like it before and it's very curious. What is it, we're not sure, but there does appear to be something there." The paper published his remarks under the dramatic headline: "US Diplomats' Brains were Shrunk by Sonic Attacks at Cuban Embassy, Study Finds" [23]. The *Washington Post* issued an editorial sarcastically titled, "Brain Trauma on the 'Friendly Island'" which claimed that a group of scientists had determined "that several dozen diplomats stationed in Havana suffered brain trauma." It asserted that the U.S. government must "demand accountability" and implied that the Cubans knew who the culprits were [31]. Some media outlets took the time to carefully weigh the evidence in the study, consulting with a range of experts. As a result, their findings were presented in a more cautious light. The *Wall Street Journal* published the subdued headline, "Slight Differences Found in Brains of Ex-Cuba Diplomats" [32]. The Voice of America was also restrained, interviewing Psychiatry Professor Sophia Frangou of the Mount Sinai Icahn School of Medicine in New York, who reviewed the claims and found them unconvincing. R. Douglas Fields of the National Institute of Health echoed her sentiments, observing that the study's main contribution to understanding the Cuban saga was what the researchers did not find. "If there'd been brain injury, that would have been evident on the clinical brain imaging studies that were done before… There was no evidence of any pathology, and these more sophisticated measures confirm that" [26]. The science editor of *The Guardian*, Ian Sample, was also cautious, writing that "the findings were not conclusive." Dr. Paul Matthews, the Head of Brain Sciences at Imperial College London, was similarly unimpressed, noting that the study was riddled with shortcomings and failed to "meet usual standards for publication, particularly in a high-profile journal." He observed that the differences were minor and did "not correspond to known patterns of brain injury" and thus "could not be shown to have changed in the people before and after the exposure… There is little that one can conclude from what is presented," he cautioned [33]. The Director of the Wellcome Trust Centre for Neuroimaging at University College London, Professor Ray Dolan, was equally dubious. "I would take the findings with a pinch of salt," he said [33].

During early July 2019, criticism of psychological explanations for the outbreak in Cuba continued as University of Toronto Psychiatry Professor Edward Shorter wrote an emotional commentary complaining that such theories were insulting to the diplomats who had served their countries, and their families. Under the title, "'Havana Syndrome' symptoms of diplomats in Cuba are not mass hysteria," he claimed that such assessments were disrespectful. "It is a disservice to the men and women of the United States and Canadian diplomatic services to suggest they are suffering from a 'mass psychogenic illness' arising from their tenure in Havana" [34]. As evidence that the patients had been the victims of some type of attack, he cited the Michael Hoffer-led study and observed that inner ear damage could not be psychogenic. When someone challenged the validity of this study, his defense was that "the Hoffer study…passed the review process of *Investigative Otolaryngology*." He then cited the 2018 *JAMA* article and noted that the investigators had uncovered "traumatic brain injuries akin to concussions." As a result, he concluded that the hysteria explanation "simply defies belief" because 'mass hysteria' cannot cause brain lesions.

Shorter *assumes* that just because peer-reviewed journals published studies claiming that there was ear and brain damage respectively, there must be merit to the claims, while failing to point out a single flaw in these studies that were riddled with flaws [34]. Over 3 months later in October 2019, we asked Dr. Shorter if he had reconsidered his position. It was unchanged. "The evidence is now overwhelming that the 'Havana Syndrome' is somatogenic (that is, it arises from physiological causes and are not psychogenic in origin). I refer you to Benedict Carey's overview of the subject in the NYT, July 23, 2019. Since then, there have been other studies…But the science now points to organicity, possibly caused by an insecticide that the Cubans sprayed liberally about the city" [35]. Shorter's reaction underscores how respected specialists, even on psychogenic illness, can be misled if they have either not read or understood the research. Shorter has taken these studies on their face value and assumed there were brain lesions and ear damage caused by some external agent, when a closer scrutiny of the evidence shows nothing of the sort.

The Canadian Fumigation Study

Attacks on the psychogenic illness explanation gained new life in September *2019, when a study funded by the Canadian government concluded that the likely culprit for the mysterious symptoms in Canadian Embassy diplomats and their families, was exposure to neurotoxins from pesticides. The researchers noted that since 2016, the Cuban government had been engaged in an aggressive public spraying campaign to control the Zika virus which is spread by mosquitoes. Zika is responsible for several neurological conditions, most notably birth defects. They wrote that their findings were consistent with "the diagnosis of acquired brain injury"* [36, p 3]. T*he study's release* was used to once again ridicule the psychogenic illness explanation, with Dr. Douglas Smith taking the opportunity to claim that the Canadian findings were vindication for the patients who were studied at the University of Pennsylvania Center for Brain Injury and Repair. He noted that his patients felt "under assault" in response to claims that they were imaginary. "People outside keep making claims that this is psychological. This might give them some peace and some vindication that there is something real there and it is not just in their heads," he said. "Everyone who examined these patients feels this was real from a neurological point of view, that this was a true neurological disorder," he asserted. Most journalists are not experts in advanced neuroimaging, and they assume that when studies are produced for government agencies or in major medical journals like *JAMA*, that the findings are sound. Hence, in the same article with Smith's interview, journalist Elizabeth Payne wrote that "the new study confirms that the diplomats and their families suffered from brain injuries." She also included the observation by Reuters journalist Alexandre Meneghini that "An early suggestion ascribing so-called 'Havana Syndrome' among diplomats to 'mass hysteria' has now been generally dismissed" [37].

A psychiatrist who was involved in the fumigation study, Cindy Calkin, told the Canadian Broadcasting Corporation that mass hysteria played no part in the symptoms. "I have interviewed all but one or two…[victims] and I haven't found any evidence of psychiatric disorder. This is a very strong group, very resilient and there is no evidence of mass hysteria." She also noted that "Part of the diagnostic of mass hysteria is that there is no underlying other medical cause that can be found. And we [found] underlying medical evidence" [38]. This statement shows a lack of understanding about psychogenic illness, suggesting that it occurs among weak-minded persons who are suffering from a mental disorder. Characterizing it as a "psychiatric disorder" is inaccurate. Mass psychogenic illness is a collective stress reaction in normal people. Despite claims of underlying medical evidence of brain trauma, there were serious problems with the study. It was speculative and poorly designed, included a range of nonspecific tests, and had no adequate control group. It had not even been peer-reviewed at the time it was released and would almost certainly fail a rigorous peer-review. There were other logical inconsistencies. For instance, how can they explain the Chinese Embassy 'sonic attacks' and health complaints? Why has there not been an epidemic of concussion-like symptoms across Cuba? While they noted that the Canadian Embassy was frequently fumigated and that "routine fumigation around and often inside the houses of Canadian diplomats may have added to extent of exposure," why weren't the many other diplomats from other embassies affected or Cubans in general? [36, p 35]. Why weren't non-diplomats who worked at both embassies affected? Finally, how do they explain the abrupt onset of symptoms associated with hearing sounds and the change in symptoms when moving from one location to another?

The Director of the Cuban panel of investigating 'Havana Syndrome,' Dr. Mitchell Valdés-Sosa was interviewed in the press and quoted as saying the fumigation claims were plausible. This has been taken to suggest that he supports the neurotoxin explanation or at least considers it likely. This is not true. We contacted Dr. Valdés-Sosa after the study appeared, and he said that while there was no convincing evidence for this position, like any good scientist, he was willing to work with the Canadians and would evaluate any new evidence that they could produce. According to Valdés-Sosa, the Cuban panel oversaw interviews with hundreds of people who lived near the affected diplomats' homes, and "all employees at the hotels where diplomats were lodged." The results were unremarkable. They were unable to identify any "increased prevalence of any of the symptoms described by the diplomats in the environment around the diplomats' living quarters. Some people with hearing loss were found, but they had hearing loss of long duration, so these were preexisting conditions. Nothing was found that would indicate a spillover of some noxious agent that was harming the diplomats. Nothing, in any of the several hundred interviewed" [39].

Another example of where the Canadian study's authors misrepresent the literature on mass psychogenic illness, is their analysis of Gulf War Illness. They note that many of the symptoms of 'Havana Syndrome' are similar to those experienced by U.S. troops who were exposed to organophosphate-based nerve agents in the Gulf War – the same ingredient used in the fumigations. They assert that similar symptoms have "not been reported in veterans returning from other military conflicts" and that stress was "not the major (or only) factor in the expression of these multi-symptom illnesses" [36, p 32]. This shows a remarkable lack of familiarity with the literature on combat syndromes, for, as we will learn in Chap. 4, the symptoms of Gulf War Illness mirror those found in veterans returning from every American conflict for more than a century. Furthermore, many studies have concluded that stress was indeed a key factor in these war-related illness clusters.

In summary, four separate retrospective patient studies have been published on the mysterious outbreak of illness among American and Canadian Embassy diplomats in Cuba; all have critical design flaws including selection of inappropriate controls, inflated conclusions, and a lack of evidence for exposure to an energy source or toxin. None of these studies adequately test the hypotheses they propose, while promoting exotic explanations that are not grounded in conventional research methodology or supported by the facts. Claims that these conditions are part of a novel clinical entity that has never been seen before are without foundation, yet their publication in scientific journals has generated a flurry of media reports suggesting that the diplomats developed brain damage after being exposed to some type of sonic device or toxin. These studies are speculative and fail to demonstrate a basic understanding of mass psychogenic illness, which is where the evidence overwhelmingly points. Furthermore, researchers on each of these study teams have publicly berated the possible role of mass psychogenic illness, noting that such explanations are invalid either because the patients were mentally fit or showed no evidence of feigning illness – assertions that show an alarming lack of understanding of the literature. Here is a summary of the four studies and their limitations:

The February 2018 *JAMA* study

- The threshold for impairment was inappropriate
- Misrepresented the concept of mass psychogenic illness
- Showed clear bias.
- Failed to share their data.

The December 2018 University of Miami Study

- Ear damage was not demonstrated
- No appropriate controls
- Just six of the affected diplomats reported headaches – a major feature of head injury, which is about the same as their unaffected housemates
- The 10 housemates who did not report symptoms, inexplicably were not tested
- Prior to the study, it was claimed that a third of patients had hearing loss; when the study came out, just two had hearing loss (and both of these predated going to Cuba).
- The authors took the mystifying decision not to use the housemates as a control group
- There was an array of symptoms suggestive of different causes; aside from dizziness, which is very common and notoriously difficult to measure, and there was little overlap in symptoms
- The idea that a 'sonic attack' could cause inner ear vestibular damage or brain damage without affecting hearing makes no sense

The July 2019 *JAMA* study

- Could not rule out the possibility that the differences with the healthy controls were from individual variation
- Twelve of those affected had pre-existing histories of concussion, compared to none in the healthy controls. This could explain the differences in the groups.
- The brain scans could only be interpreted with complex computer programs that have a high rate of false positives
- They conflate brain changes with brain damage

The May 2019 Canadian Fumigation Study

- Extremely speculative and preliminary; limited to observational data
- When first released to the public, it had not even been peer reviewed
- Does not explain the Chinese embassy 'attacks'
- Why has there not been an epidemic of concussion-like symptoms across Cuba?
- Cannot explain why non-diplomats working in the embassies were not affected?
- The authors assert that similar symptoms were reported in Gulf War veterans who were exposed to nerve agents but have "not been reported in veterans returning from other military conflicts," and stress is not thought to be a major factor in combat syndromes. Both claims are not supported by the literature.
- Cannot account for the differences in the Canadian and American illness experience

Mixing of Politics and Science

The articles in the *Journal of the American Medical Association* served to fuel the belief that American diplomats suffered traumatic brain injury from some mysterious energy source. These studies garnered international headlines. Many people may find it difficult to believe that such a prestigious publication could allow not one but two studies to slip through the peer-review process with serious flaws. But the history of science is replete with examples of lapses in editorial judgement in all fields. One prominent example occurred in 1991 when *JAMA* published an article extolling the benefits of Transcendental Meditation [40]. The article was rife with pseudoscientific claims. Former *JAMA* Associate editor Andrew Skolnick later wrote an exposé on the episode and noted that one of the studies cited in the article, "purported to show that a group of yogic fliers in Israel was able to reduce the level of violence in war-torn Lebanon." Skolnick cites another *JAMA* editor as admitting that despite the best laid plans, occasionally, "shoddy science" ends up being published in respected journals [41, p 257, 42]. The Cuban mystery illness is another such example.

Once the administration of US President Donald Trump first identified the illness cluster in February 2016 and defined it as a resumption of Cold War hostilities, its Cuban diplomats were counseled on the "mysterious threat" that was causing colleagues to fall ill [43]. This created further uncertainty and anxiety. Word of the 'attacks' quickly spread through the diplomatic community, resulting in several foreign embassies testing their employees for possible exposure. This could explain why some staff at the Canadian Embassy reported feeling unwell from the 'attacks.' It is conspicuous that Cubans working with American diplomats and their neighbors did not experience symptoms. Counseling staff over the perceived threat created an expectation of illness and a new frame through which to interpret future sounds and symptoms. The handling of the outbreak by the US government has exacerbated the episode due to its contradictory claims, and the use of ambiguous, dramatic descriptions such as "brain trauma," and the failure to release Freedom of Information documents or redacted medical records of those affected. The vague character of the symptoms and the attributed cause (sound) are conducive to the mechanism of contagion because the symptoms can arise from several clinical conditions including tinnitus, while sounds are common in the environment. Publicity surrounding the events has served to reaffirm, magnify and propagate the suggestive effect.

The State Department revealed the existence of the 'attacks' on August 9, 2017. Since then, the administration has expelled several Cuban diplomats serving in the US as retaliation. While they cannot prove an association between the illness cluster and agents of the Cuban government, they based their action on the grounds that Cuban officials had failed to protect foreign diplomats under the Vienna Convention [44]. On October 16, US President Trump heightened political tensions by asserting: "I do believe Cuba is responsible, yes" [45]. The ranking members of the Senate Intelligence Committee have urged the administration to "declare all accredited Cuban diplomats in the United States persona non grata" and close the American Embassy in Cuba, unless "the harassment and acoustic attacks" ceased [46, 47].

Psychogenic illness has stoked political tensions in the past. In 1983, nearly 1000 mostly Arab schoolgirls in the disputed Israeli-occupied West Bank, were reportedly poisoned by Jewish agents, prompting the United Nations to pass a resolution condemning the 'attack' and threats of war. Symptoms included fainting, headache, abdominal pain, blurred vision, and muscle weakness. Three separate investigations concluded that the outbreak was psychogenic in nature, triggered by odor from a school latrine [48, 49] and fueled by inaccurate media reports [50]. During political unrest in Soviet Georgia in 1989, Russian authorities used a noxious gas to disperse a political rally. Soon after, about 400 adolescent females in several schools near the incident, experienced abdominal pain, burning eyes, skin irritation, and dry throat amid rumors that they had been exposed to the same gas. Media coverage was instrumental in the spread of symptoms, which mimicked those of the poison gas [51]. In 1990, an illness outbreak among at least 4000 residents in the Serbian province of Kosovo triggered an outbreak of pseudo-poisonings involving headache, dizziness, hyperventilation, weakness, burning sensations, cramps, chest pain, nausea, and dry mouth. The episode was triggered by ethnic tension between Serbs and Albanians and was fueled by rumors, the scrutinization of mundane odors and substances, and mass communications. The dramatic proliferation of cases across the province on March 22, coincided with the implementation of an emergency disaster plan whereby ethnic Albanians had seized control of public health services [52].

Humans are curious creatures. Time and again throughout history, groups of people have come to believe in the existence of the most fantastic things, without evidence to support those beliefs. Often the consequences are tragic. During the Middle Ages, the belief in witches and demons led to the execution of upwards of half a million people who were suspected of consorting with the Devil. In our modern society, we often feel shielded from such beliefs. The ignorant and gullible from the Middle Ages may have fallen for it, but certainly not in today's modern, educated society. Nothing could be further from the truth. One of the poignant lessons from this book is how easily people living today – as in the past – are susceptible to being led astray from objective reality, especially when it comes to arcane topics where only a few people have the expertise and the so-called experts have presented flawed research. 'Havana Syndrome' is one such episode.

This story has all the elements of a good spy novel that is part comedy, part tragedy. The comic aspect is that some of the key players in triggering the episode, were lovelorn insects. As for the tragedy, the episode has cost millions in taxpayer dollars and harmed dozens of people, caused undue alarm, and led to a major diplomatic row between two longtime enemies who were just getting on track for a new era in thawing relations after decades of Cold War tension. The case of the sonic attack on US Embassy staff in Cuba is an extraordinary tale of bad science, political ineptitude, public confusion, and the nature of the media which is prone to promoting false narratives because most journalists, like the general public, are not experts on exotic and highly specialized subjects like neuro-weapons. But above all, this is a story about life in the early twenty-first century in the era of conspiracy theories and fake news. What is the public to believe when faced with competing stories by experts and how do we determine the truth? Historically, when claims are in dispute, people have turned to science and scientists as the arbitrator of truth. But in the case of the 'sonic attack,' many scientists have muddied the waters with the publication of flawed studies that lack evidence to support their claims. In many instances they have been aided and abetted by media outlets. The Cuban history of harassing American diplomatic staff in Havana laid the foundation for the wave of 'attacks' that were to come. So, when the first patients began reporting symptoms and associating noises with them, there was an assumption by a politically paranoid Trump administration that the Cubans must be involved. It turned into a self-fulfilling prophesy and is reminiscent of the words of Shakespeare's *A Midsummer Night's Dream*: "Or in the night, imagining some fear, How easy is a bush supposed a bear!" Perhaps this should be updated to read: "How easy is a cricket or cicada supposed a sonic attack!"

References

1. Smith M. Canadian children were among those affected by sonic attacks in Cuba, documents suggest. National Post (Toronto). 4 Jan 2018.
2. Campion-Smith B. Brain-injured diplomats feel 'abandoned' by Ottawa. Toronto Star. 2 July 2018.
3. Campion-Smith B. Canadian and American diplomats in Cuba hit by 'directed energy,' U.S. doctor says. Toronto Star. 20 Apr 2018.

4. Wolde-Giorghis A. Diplomats sue Ottawa for $28M over health ailments during Cuba postings. Canadian Broadcasting Corporation. 8 Feb 2019.
5. Fox K. Canadian diplomats sue their government over mystery illness in Cuba. CNN News (Atlanta, GA). 7 Feb 2019.
6. Canada reducing staff at Cuba embassy by half following latest illness. The Sun (Lowell, MA). 31 Jan 2019.
7. Canadian Federal Court File Number T-238-19, filed February 6, 2019, in Toronto, Canada between the plaintiffs and Her Majesty the Queen in Right of Canada, Ontario Regional Office, Department of Justice Canada, 120 Adelaide Street West, Suite #400, Toronto, accepted by Mavis Griffith, Senior Registry Officer, Agent principal du greffe, p. 4.
8. Pelley S. Brain damage suffered by U.S. diplomats abroad could be work of hostile foreign government. 60 Minutes (CBS News, NY). 17 Mar 2019.
9. Fields, RD. CBS 60 Minutes sensationalized report on a sonic or microwave weapon harming US diplomats. 2019 Mar 21. https://rdouglasfields.com/2019/03/cbs-60-minutes-sensationalized-report-on-a-sonic-or-microwave-weapon-harming-us-diplomats/. Accessed 7 May 2019.
10. Oppmann P, Koran L. Senate holds hearing on Cuba 'sonic attacks.' CNN. 9 Jan 2018.
11. Fields RD. The Cuban 'sonic attack' and journalist ethics. Sci Am. 18 Mar 2019.
12. de Granados O, Rey M. 60 Minutes overtime inside the story. 2019 Mar 17. https://www.youtube.com/watch?v=YBdFM8AuHk8&t=7s. Accessed 15 Nov.
13. Muth C, Lewis SL. Editorial: neurological symptoms among US diplomats in Cuba. JAMA. 2018;319(11):1098–1100 (March 20). https://doi.org/10.1001/jama.2018.1780.
14. Bartholomew RE. Neurological symptoms in US government personnel In Cuba. Letter. JAMA. 2018;320(6):602 (August 14). https://doi.org/10.1001/jama.2018.8702.
15. Stone J, Popkirov S, Carson AJ. Letter. JAMA. 2018;320(6):602–3 (August 14). https://doi.org/10.1001/jama.2018.8706.
16. Shura RD, Kacmarski JA, Miskey HM. Letter. JAMA. 2018;320(6):603 (August 14). https://doi.org/10.1001/jama.2018.8698.
17. Gianoli JG. Soileau JS, Wackym PA. Letter. JAMA 2018;320(6):603–4 (August 14). https://doi.org/10.1001/jama.2018.8713.
18. Ragini V, Swanson, RL, Parker D, Ismail A, Shinohara RT, Alappatt JA, et al. Neuroimaging findings in US government personnel with possible exposure to directional phenomena in Havana, Cuba. JAMA. 2019;322(4):336–47 (July 23). https://doi.org/10.1001/jama.2019.9269. See p. 336.
19. Diplomat brain hell. The Sun (London). 25 July 2019. p. 23.
20. Steinbuch Y. Cuba 'sonic attacks' changed US diplomats' brains, study finds. The New York Post. 23 July 2019.
21. Scully R. Brain scans hint the mysterious 'sonic attack' in Cuba was real. New Scientist. 23 July 2019.
22. Scans show changes to brains of 'injured' Havana U.S. embassy workers. Reuters. 24 July 2019.
23. US diplomats' brains were shrunk by sonic attacks at Cuban embassy, study finds. The Daily Telegraph. 23 July 2019.
24. Stone is an accomplished neurologist, but his views on mass psychogenic illness are extreme. He told *The New York Times Magazine* that he is opposed to the term in part because of the public perception that it creates – that the symptoms are purely psychological. "I wince when I hear the word 'psychogenic,'" as it generates "a false impression about what these disorders are," suggesting that it is 'all in their heads.' "The term 'mass hysteria' is just ridiculous and insulting," he said. He believes that presenting the Cuban outbreaks as 'mass hysteria' is unlikely to persuade the public at-large, whereas presenting the problem as everyday symptoms and illnesses which are common in the general population, is more helpful. This position fails to adequately address the social and cultural context and framing of the Havana illness through rumors, social networks, work channels, and media reports, and the powerful role of the nocebo effect. See Hurley D. The diplomat's disorder. The New York Times Magazine. 19 May 2019, p. 40–5, 71.

25. Eklund A, Nichols TE, Knutsson H. Cluster failure: why fMRI inferences for spatial extent have inflated false-positive rates. PNAS USA. 2016;113:7900–5. Erratum in Proc Natl Acad Sci USA 113:E4929.

26. Hamilton J. Injury in U.S. diplomats who fell ill in Cuba. All Things Considered (Washington DC). National public radio broadcast airing on 23 July 2019.

27. What was needed was a careful epidemiological study that focuses on the patients and unaffected cohorts, the timing and progression of symptoms, standardized tests and search for any possible exposures including stress and negative expectations. To date, there is no credible evidence that their symptoms resulted from some type of attack.

28. Whipple T. US envoys in Cuba have brain damage. The Times (London). 24 July 2019. p. 33.

29. Hess P. Brain imaging of US diplomats rules out leading theory on 'Havana syndrome.' Inverse. 2019 Jul 23. https://www.inverse.com/article/57924-what-caused-the-havana-syndrome-in-us-diplomats. Accessed 19 Oct 2019.

30. Payne E. 'Not just in their heads:' scientists find anomalies in brains of 'Havana syndrome' patients. Ottawa Citizen. 29 Sept 2019.

31. Brain trauma on the 'friendly island.' The Washington Post. 27 July 2019;Sect. A:16.

32. Abbott B. Slight differences found in brains of ex-Cuba diplomats. The Wall Street Journal. 23 July 2019.

33. Sample I. Brain scans of US embassy staff to Cuba may show abnormalities. The Guardian. 23 July 2019.

34. Shorter E. 'Havana syndrome' symptoms of diplomats in Cuba are not mass hysteria. The Conversation. 4 July 2019.

35. Letter from Edward Shorter to Robert Bartholomew, 21 Oct 2019.

36. Friedman A, Calkin C, Adams A, Suarez G, Bardouille T, Hacohen N, Green A, et al. Havana syndrome among Canadian diplomats: brain imaging reveals acquired neurotoxicity. Research report, Brain Repair Centre, Dalhousie University, Life Sciences Research Institute, Halifax, Nova Scotia, Canada; 2019, 48pp.

37. Payne E. Canadian research points to pesticides as possible cause of Havana syndrome. The Ottawa Citizen. 24 Sept 2019.

38. Chartrand L, Movilla M, Ellenwood L. Havana syndrome: exposure to neurotoxin may have been cause, study Suggests. CBC (Canadian Broadcasting Corporation) News. 29 Sept 2019.

39. Reed G. What happened to the US diplomats in Havana? Mitchell Valdés MD PhD Director, Cuban Neuroscience Center. Int J Cuban Health Med. 2018;20(4):14–9.

40. Sharma HM, Brihaspati DT, Chopra D. Letter from New Delhi. Maharishi Ayur-Veda: modern insights into ancient medicine. JAMA. 1991;265(20):2633–7. (May 22–29)

41. Skolnick A. The Maharishi caper: JAMA hoodwinked (but just for a while). Skept Inq. 1992;16(3):254–9. See p 257

42. Skolnick A. Maharishi Ayur-Veda: Guru's marketing scheme promises the world eternal 'perfect health'. JAMA. 1991;266(13):1741–50.

43. Oppmann P, Labott E. US diplomats, families in Cuba targeted nearly 50 times by sonic attacks, says US official. CNN News. 23 Sept 2017.

44. Nauert H. US Department of State press briefing. 9 Aug 2017.

45. Nauert H. US Department of State press briefing. 17 Oct 2017.

46. Rubio M. US Senator (FL), press release. 15 Sept 2017.

47. Zengerle P. Frank M. U.S. lawmakers want retaliation for sonic attacks in Cuba. Reuters. 16 Sept 2017.

48. Modan B, Tirosh M, Weissenberg E, Acker C, Swartz T, Costin C, et al. The Arjenyattah epidemic. Lancet. 1983;2:1472–4.

49. Landrigan PJ, Miller B. The Arjenyattah epidemic: home interview data and toxicological aspects. Lancet. 1983;2:1474–6.

50. Hafez A. The role of the press and the medical community in an epidemic of mysterious gas poisoning in the Jordan West Bank. Am J Psych. 1985;142:833–7.

51. Goldsmith M. Physicians with Georgia on their minds. JAMA. 1989;262:603–4.

52. Radovanovic Z. On the origin of mass casualty incidents in Kosovo, Yugoslavia, in 1990. Eur J Epidemiol. 1996;12:101–13.

Psychogenic Illness on the Battlefield: From the Civil War to Gulf War Syndrome

4

Post-combat syndromes have arisen after all major wars over the past century, and we can predict that they will continue to appear after future conflicts. What cannot be accurately forecast is their form, as they are moulded by the changing nature of health fears and warfare. …each new post-combat syndrome is…part of an understandable pattern of normal responses to the physical and psychological stress of war…

–Edgar Jones [1, p 5]

During every major American conflict since the Civil War, doctors have noticed clusters of unexplained symptoms in soldiers who were exposed to traumatic events. After undergoing thorough exams, they were unable to pinpoint a cause. There is a growing consensus in the medical community that the fear and uncertainty that accompanies these events give rise to outbreaks of psychogenic illness. These episodes typically involve the appearance of persistent neurological symptoms that can and have been misdiagnosed as concussions and brain damage. This is directly relevant to the situation in Cuba because the diplomats who became sick were essentially participants in a continuation of the Cold War, living in a hostile foreign country where they knew their every move was being closely watched. There was also a lengthy and well-documented history of Embassy staff suffering harassment at the hands of Cuban agents. They soon began to hear alarming stories of sonic attacks. New staff were not only being briefed on the likelihood that they may become the next targets, they were played recordings of the sounds captured by employees on the ground in Havana, before taking up their posts – sounds that were later identified as crickets and cicadas. As a result, between late 2016 and much of 2017, staff in Havana were living in a cauldron of stress and uncertainty. They were not being targeted by bullets and bombs; their enemy was silent and invisible as they worried that they may be the victims of an enigmatic new weapon. As one worker who lived through this ordeal told us, they were afraid to even retire to their beds at night, fearful that they and their families would be attacked in their sleep. There was no respite and no place to hide.

© Springer Nature Switzerland AG 2020
R. W. Baloh, R. E. Bartholomew, *Havana Syndrome*,
https://doi.org/10.1007/978-3-030-40746-9_4

Even before modern doctors began closely monitoring the health of soldiers involved in modern warfare and on their return from the battlefield, history books were filled with accounts of unexplained symptoms after exposure to wartime trauma. In writing about the battle of Marathon in 490 B.C., the Greek historian Herodotus told of an Athenian soldier who suddenly lost his sight after seeing a comrade who was standing next to him, killed in battle [2]. Similar accounts are common in the annals of military history and were later referred to as hysterical blindness. A kindred condition known as 'nostalgia' was identified by Swiss doctors in 1678 as it included intense homesickness along with depression, weakness, insomnia, palpitations and stupor [2]. During the *Napoleonic Wars* of the early nineteenth century, unexplained symptoms appeared in soldiers who were traumatized after narrowly escaping death from projectiles whizzing by them or being in the vicinity of an explosion but were physically unharmed. The condition was given the name 'wind contusions' or 'cerebrospinal shock' [3].

The U.S. Civil War

During the American Civil War many traumatized soldiers began to present with outward signs of heart disease, yet the typical exam yielded no cardiac problems and patients seemed to be in good overall health. Symptoms included breathlessness after minor exertion, chest pain, palpitations, rapid pulse, headache, dizziness, exhaustion, insomnia, vision problems, and giddiness. The condition was given such labels as soldier's heart and effort syndrome. The physician who made these observations, Jacob Da Costa, surmised that there were similar conditions among the civilian population [4]. Some physicians of the period saw parallels with other conditions that were attributed to trauma, but there was no apparent physical cause, such as with 'railway spine.' Soon after the advent of rail transportation, passengers who had survived serious train accidents began to complain of a variety of health issues including back pain, difficulty walking, abnormal eye movements, unusual sensations in the limbs, insomnia, fatigue, sluggishness, confusion, and visual impairment. Doctors initially attributed these symptoms to "spinal concussion" resulting from the crash. However, it soon became apparent that, like effort syndrome, they were looking at stressed patients with an array of unexplained symptoms. This led some doctors to conclude that the same mysterious condition seen in the Civil War soldiers, was masquerading as 'railway spine' [5]. Their position was bolstered in 1883, when London Surgeon Herbert Page established "that in many cases no damage had been sustained to the spinal cord," which led him to conclude that "fright alone" led to the symptoms [3, p 12].

The First World War

During World War I, a 'new' condition was identified called shell shock, the symptoms of which bear a striking similarity with those experienced by the American diplomats in Cuba – right down to the claims of concussion-like symptoms. As one of the *JAMA* study authors, Dr. Randel Swanson remarked: "It's like a concussion without a concussion [6]. Curiously, during the First World War, many soldiers who had not seen direct action, and hence, with no obvious combat-related cause for their symptoms such as an exploding shell or bullet wound, were initially diagnosed with *concussion-like symptoms*. It was only after a more careful review of the data was it realized that what they were seeing was an epidemic of psychogenic illness. While the condition was common during the American Civil War, this figure paled in comparison to the number of soldiers who were diagnosed with shell shock in World War I. While many more troops were involved in the war and there was a more thorough scrutiny of medical records, there was also a dramatic increase in artillery firepower. For instance, an estimated half million shells were fired by the French Army over a 5-day period during the battle on the Marne, east of Paris in September 1914. In just 50 seconds, the field guns could spray an area equivalent to ten acres, pocking the ground with a patchwork of massive craters [7]. On top of that, political and military leaders were stubbornly willing to expose millions of men to this devastating barrage without any end-goal in sight. Imagine crouching in a foxhole, day after day, hearing a sound like the roar of an express train barreling overhead, wondering when and where it will burst? An American Red Cross worker described the impact from an exploding shell: "It was terrible. The concussion felt like a blow in the face, the stomach and all over; it was like being struck unexpectedly by a huge wave in the ocean" [8]. Remarkably, the shell had exploded 200 yards away. Of the estimated 9.7 million military fatalities during the war, about 60 percent were shrapnel injuries from mortars and artillery shells. The sounds of whizzing artillery shells and their terrorizing effects struck fear into soldiers on both sides of the war. As a result, several million suffered from shell shock, a psychogenic illness caused by experiencing or hearing about the carnage associated with this terrible war [9].

The term shell shock was first used by Captain Charles Myers of the Royal Army Medical Corps in an article in the English medical journal *The Lancet* in February 1915 [10]. Myers, who trained in psychology at Cambridge University, described three soldiers who had suffered from major blast injuries. One was catapulted into the air by a nearby explosion; another was buried underground for 18 hours after a shell exploded next to his foxhole, and the third witnessed several nearby explosions. These soldiers had a range of neurological and psychological complaints: some had lost their sense of smell and taste or had memory impairment, all of which could be reasonably attributed to brain concussion. Thus, the initial use of the term shell shock was for a physical brain injury that merited an honorable discharge and potential war pension. But by early 1916, it became apparent that many soldiers were experiencing similar symptoms but had not been near an exploding shell. At first, doctors were baffled. They appeared to be suffering from a concussion without a concussion. Symptoms included trembling and shaking, paralysis, vison loss, ringing in the ears, dizziness, headache, confusion, difficulty concentrating, loss of memory and impaired sleep. In some soldiers, it was obvious that the symptoms were due to brain trauma such as the initial three cases described in the *The Lancet* article, but in many others, most of the symptoms had no clear cause. The term shell shock soon became an all-encompassing label used for all direct combat injuries, and soldiers who did not experience such physical trauma. Myers would later describe many of the symptoms of shell shock as functional or non-organic, meaning that they had no apparent physical cause [11].

Shell shock posed a challenge for doctors of the day just as the array of similar symptoms in Cuba has created modern-day controversy and confusion within the medical community. During both periods, there was no dearth of opinions to explain the symptoms associated with the diagnosis. Once the *JAMA* team had published their findings in early 2018, there was a swift response by specialists who pointed out the obvious psychogenic features of the outbreak. During the Great War, faced with accumulating evidence that the affected soldiers had not been subjected to exploding ordinance, some doctors continued to suggest that sufferers must have had subtle microscopic brain tears or hemorrhages that had been triggered by the blast waves, but once they had a chance to analyze the data, a pattern began to take shape and a consensus emerged that traumatic stress and suggestibility were the root of most cases. The mind had become debilitated by emotional trauma and fear. Over time, many European neurologists and psychiatrists concluded that shell shock had a psychological origin. The chief consultant in psychiatry with the American Expeditionary Forces in France, Thomas Salmon pointed out that soldiers' symptoms often mirrored their wartime experiences. This is a longstanding feature and telltale sign of psychogenic illness [12]. In some cases, soldiers developed blindness after witnessing a traumatic event or became deaf after hearing unbearable cries for help from wounded comrades. Of course, there were still those who thought that the soldiers were fabricating their symptoms to get out of harm's way and that they deserved harsh treatment rather than sympathy and a discharge. How the affected soldiers were treated changed during the war and varied dramatically from country to country.

In late 1915, the British Army Council instructed doctors who were treating men with nervous or mental symptoms to separate them into two categories. The first was for those who appeared to be suffering from physical wounds. They were labeled 'shell shock W' for wounded. The second category was for suspected psychogenic trauma who were given the label 'shell shock S' for sick [13]. It quickly became apparent that these decisions were being arbitrarily made at the front. A better system was needed. By 1917, a new category was devised: NYDN or Not Yet Diagnosed Nervous. Soldiers with this label were transferred to treatment centers. The goal was to get them back to the battlefield as soon as possible. The result was disastrous. Some soldiers with shell shock were found wandering about and were shot on the spot for desertion. Some of the most severely affected were transferred to the National Neurological Hospital in London [14]. Examples include a 23-year-old private who developed a feeling of worms crawling in his lower abdomen, shortness of breath, dizzy spells, sleeplessness, a sensation of choking, and general weakness. These symptoms appeared after a shell exploded in a nearby trench and witnessing other traumatic events. Many soldiers developed symptoms away from the battlefield, while on leave or after being discharged. Neurologists used a variety of terms to describe the psychological trauma they were suffering from: functional disorder, hysteria, neurasthenia, neurosis, and shell shock. A kindred condition was called 'gas hysteria,' which was used to describe soldiers who had minimal exposure to chemical weapons such as phosgene or chlorine gas and completely recovered yet suffered from chronic ill-health [5].

Mass psychogenic illness has been notoriously difficult to diagnose due to the range of symptoms it can produce, especially when they first appear, as they often reflect specific scenarios. For instance, a soldier who erroneously believes that he has been sprayed with toxic gas may experience itchy, watery eyes, skin rash and headache. Once other conditions have been eliminated, and in the absence of an underlying organic cause, the diagnosis becomes apparent. As a group, those with shell shock could be described as suffering from an array of neurological abnormalities that did not fit any known condition. US Embassy staff in Cuba were also suffering from abnormal neurological findings. As with the Cuban saga, soon after the first diagnosis of shell shock, doctors initially went on a wild goose chase trying to find a reason for the abnormalities such as brain damage. Before long, the diagnosis of 'shell shock' became passé and the term functional disorder soon took its place. This refers to problems in the way that the overstimulated nervous system and the body function to send and receive signals. The most common treatments used at the London Neurological Hospital were electrotherapy (electric shocks) combined with re-education, suggestion, and physical therapy using massage, baths, heat, and exercise. While this may sound humane and relaxing, it was anything but. A soldier with a paralyzed arm was not asked but *ordered* to raise it and if he did not, the arm was repeatedly shocked until he did so. A patient who was mute received shocks to his throat and *ordered* to speak. The shocks were repeated for hours until he began to stammer and cry [15].

Near the end of the war, many neurologists began to hypothesize that shell shock was a malfunction of brain physiology caused by prolonged stress. Harvard researcher, Walter Cannon, discovered that stress triggered the release of hormones such as adrenalin linking emotions and adrenaline to the production of psychogenic symptoms. In 1915, he coined the term "fight or flight," which were the only two options available for primitive prey in the face of a predator [16]. Fear and stress could activate neurons in the hypothalamus, stimulating the release of multiple hormones including adrenalin. An injection of adrenalin, in turn, could result in shaking, agitation, palpitations, sweating, shortness of breath, nausea, abdominal pain, near-faint dizziness, ringing in the ears and difficulty concentrating – all symptoms common in psychogenic illness. To explain psychogenic paralysis and fits, neurologists turned to Hughling Jackson's evolutionary model of brain development where more primitive emotional and reflex centers were under the cognitive control of the more advanced cortical centers. Breakdown in these cognitive control centers due to prolonged emotional stress could result in the expression of primitive emotions and behaviors.

World War II and Traumatic Neurosis

During the Second World War, emotional responses to the trauma of war in American soldiers were known by a variety of names ranging from 'combat fatigue,' 'battle fatigue,' and 'combat stress reaction.' At the start of the war, American military brass did not assign psychiatrists to combat divisions because they believed they could screen out potential problem patients. In Britain, Winston Churchill even sent a memorandum to his War Council asking them to restrict the activities of psychiatrists and psychologists as much as possible as they tend to ask 'odd' questions that might disturb healthy men and women [17]. But, as with previous wars, clusters of unexplained symptoms began to appear. The variety of psychiatric symptoms reported by soldiers in the Second World War were similar to those in the First World War but there was a trend away from paralysis and fits, towards more subtle symptoms such as blurred vision, dizziness and hearing problems, a trend that was also noticed in the civilian population [18]. It was not uncommon for the symptom profile to fit the soldier's type of field duty. For example, members of the air force would develop blurring of vision, impaired depth perception or diminished night vision that would disqualify them from flying but otherwise not be disabling. A sharpshooter might have blurry vision in just his shooting eye [18].

Another feature of the war were deliberate attacks on civilian populations, which far exceeded the number of military deaths. Civilians were also exposed to massive shelling and bombing, unlike anything in previous wars. Initially, the British government came to the remarkable conclusion that overall civilian mental health had improved during the war! This was attributed to their being so busy playing their roles in keeping society going that they had no time for illness. Overall, patients with psychiatric symptoms were largely ignored since the governments were focusing their resources on the military and it was in their best interest to paint a picture of a healthy population doing their part in the war effort. Hospitals and clinics were understaffed and patients quickly learned that they provided little help. However, the delayed effects of war stress affected a large part of the population and resulted in a wide range of symptoms in later years.

After World War II, American psychiatrists Roy Grinker and John Spiegel provided a detailed description of 65 soldiers with psychogenic illnesses in their 1945 book, *Men and Stress* [19]. They separated acute symptoms occurring in combat from delayed symptoms developing after combat. The appearance of delayed psychogenic illness was called 'war neurosis.' This condition included psychosomatic states, depression, aggressive and hostile reactions, and even psychotic-like states. This set the stage for what later would become post-traumatic stress disorder or PTSD. More than 40 years after the Second World War, the French psychiatrists, Marc-Antoine and Louis Crocq studied a group of French citizens in the Alsace-Lorraine region at the beginning of the War. They had been conscripted by the Germans and then held captive in a Russian prison camp [20]. Of the 525 former soldiers interviewed with questionnaires, 82 percent still had vivid recollections and nightmares of their war-time experiences, 73 percent had to try hard not to think about the trauma they endured, and 40 percent continued to have survivor guilt. Political and social factors unique to the Alsace-Lorraine region explain the remarkably high rate of psychogenic symptoms. Citizens of the region speak French and German and had cultural roots in both countries. They had been forced to fight for the Germans to save their families yet were treated as Germans when captured by the Russians. When repatriated after the war, the French people who had their own guilt issues from the early surrender to the Germans, could not forgive them for fighting with the Germans. Throughout the history of war, political and social intrigue are major factors in the development of psychogenic symptoms.

The Korean and Vietnam Wars

During the Korean Conflict, once again clusters of unexplained symptoms appeared among British and American soldiers and were given such labels as 'battle fatigue' and 'combat exhaustion' in Commonwealth troops. While the incidence was reported to have been low, a re-examination of the medical records of one combat division suggests that cases were "intentionally underreported." In his study of Korean medical records, historian Edgar Jones suggests that psychogenic illness may have appeared in the form of injuries that were attributed to the cold temperatures. He writes that "Psychiatrists in Korea observed that as the incidence of frostbite increased, the number of psychiatric casualties decreased" [21]. In the Vietnam War, clusters of unexplained symptoms that were associated with trauma were given the name post-Vietnam syndrome and later post-traumatic stress disorder or PTSD for short. The percentage of soldiers with delayed combat effects including psychosomatic symptoms and substance abuse was relatively high compared to other wars. It was estimated that a quarter of all Vietnam veterans required some type of psychological intervention [20]. PTSD consisted of flashbacks and dreams of the distressing combat event; loss of emotion and avoidance of situations reminiscent of the traumatic event; and a constant state of arousal [22]. There was also a considerable overlap with symptoms of earlier wars including fatigue, shortness of breath, headaches, memory problems, trouble concentrating, muscle and joint pains, insomnia, lightheadedness, palpitations and chest pains.

Concussion-Like Symptoms in Afghanistan and Iraq

With more recent wars there has been a renewed interest in the role of traumatic brain injury in post-traumatic stress disorders. As with shell shock in World War I, soldiers exposed to explosions suffered a range of symptoms from memory loss and amnesia to anxiety and depression. At the same time, some troops developed symptoms after a blast without losing consciousness and may have suffered from mild traumatic brain injury. These are injuries that are severe enough to cause symptoms without obvious neurological findings. Many soldiers returning from Afghanistan and Iraq complained of a range of symptoms including memory impairment, dizziness and imbalance, headaches, and difficulty with decision-making [23]. While some of these soldiers suffered concussions associated with roadside explosions, others were not close enough to be concussed. Like shell shock in World War I, many of the seemingly concussed soldiers were nowhere near an explosion when their symptoms began and their complaints persisted for months or years [24]. While some patients could be feigning symptoms, most medical experts agree that faking symptoms is relatively rare when dealing with post-traumatic symptoms of psychogenic origin [25].

The Persian Gulf War

Soldiers in the 1990–1991 Gulf War suffered the same types of psychogenic symptoms and illnesses as their comrades from earlier twentieth century wars. The clustering of unexplained symptoms in this cohort became known as Gulf War Syndrome. In August 1990, in response to the invasion of Kuwait by Saddam Hussein, the United States led a coalition of United Nation troops to invade Iraq and remove Hussein's forces from Kuwait. The war was brief and successful, with relatively few casualties on the UN side. A negotiated settlement ended the war in February 1991. Most of the nearly 700,000 American troops who were sent to the Gulf did not fight in the brief war but were crowded for months in tents and storage buildings in extreme desert heat, not knowing when they would return home. About a fifth of US forces were National Guard troops who did not even expect to leave the United States. Soldiers were under constant stress with rumors of the likely use of chemical and biological weapons. Many had to wear bulky protection suits not designed for the desert heat. There was frightening gossip of dangerous side-effects from vaccines and medications given them to protect against nerve gas and deadly microbes such as Anthrax. Many of the soldiers were exposed to the smoke of burning oil wells, while others were nearby when arsenals of chemical weapons were blown up [26].

When these soldiers finally returned home, many of them began complaining of everything from aches and pains and severe fatigue to rashes and diarrhea. Some had typical symptoms of fibromyalgia and chronic fatigue syndrome, illnesses endemic in the civilian population that are suspected to have a psychosomatic genesis, while others appeared to be suffering from typical symptoms of PTSD. Some of the veterans reported bizarre symptoms such as bleeding from their gums and penis, which was quickly lumped under a new convenient label. Two veterans in Mississippi actually claimed that their penises were shrinking! [27] The majority of soldiers felt that Gulf War Syndrome was a new and unique illness; many thought it was contagious and could be passed to others. Wives and other family members came down with similar symptoms months after the soldiers returned home. Some wives were convinced that the illness could be sexually transmitted and even caused birth defects in their newborns. One partner reported that her husband's semen was toxic and caused "blisters which actually open and bleed" [28, p 116]. Although most doctors were baffled by the illnesses, some physicians and most of the veterans were sure it was caused by a toxin or infectious disease acquired while serving in the Gulf.

While many Vietnam veterans were accepting of the PTSD diagnosis as an explanation for chronic symptoms upon returning home, most Gulf War veterans were openly hostile to the diagnosis. An English nurse who developed chronic fatigue several months after her husband returned from the Gulf War argued: "This can't be psychological. I've spoken to too many veterans whose families are suffering similar symptoms" [29, p 135]. An African American veteran from Alabama who couldn't leave his house due to severe anxiety and insomnia, angrily told a journalist: "Post traumatic stress, my black ass" [29, p 135]. Self-help groups formed by Gulf War veterans and their families outright rejected the possibility of psychological illness and many blamed government agencies for covering up toxic and infectious causes to deprive them of appropriate disability payments. To the contrary, the American and British government responses to the concept of Gulf War Syndrome was overall supportive. Politicians did not want to be perceived as hostile to veterans and elected officials went out of their way not to alienate large constituencies. The seemingly ambivalent response from the United States government reinforced conspiracy rumors about the syndrome.

Numerous studies of Gulf War veterans have failed to find evidence of a unique Gulf War Syndrome or a toxic or infectious cause for the symptoms. A study of over a thousand sick Gulf War veterans found that 60 percent had illnesses with identifiable causes that were not disproportionate to the random occurrence in the general population. Another 25 percent had clear psychogenic illnesses such as PTSD and depression, and the remaining 15 percent had other symptoms with no apparent cause including headaches, memory loss, fatigue, gastrointestinal issues, and insomnia – complaints that are common in patients with psychogenic illnesses. The National Academy of Sciences supported a massive survey of 18,924 veterans at a cost of $80 million. They concluded that there was "no single cause or mystery ailment to support suspicions about the existence of a Gulf War Syndrome" [29, p 137]. In England, the Royal College of Physicians reviewed the various studies of illnesses in Gulf War veterans and reached a similar conclusion, stating that "there was no single cause for the variety of illnesses suffered by the servicemen and women who have been examined" [29, p 137]. About 15 percent of the 697,000 United States troops who served in the Gulf War reported symptoms of Gulf War Syndrome whereas only about 1 percent of the 45,000 British soldiers and about 0.5 percent of the 25,000 French troops reported symptoms. Some have suggested that the low rate in the French troops may have been from not receiving the cocktail of drugs and vaccines that were given the British and American troops, but this would not explain the disparity between the Americans and British.

Reports of Gulf War Syndrome continued to be reported at about the same rate with the second Gulf War in 2003, and the Afghan War which began in October 2001 in response to the September 11 terror attacks of the same year. Given the lack of evidence for a unique syndrome, the US Department of Veterans Affairs refers to the symptoms as "medically unexplained illnesses." Between 2010 and 2015, the Veteran's Administration approved only about 15 percent of claims for health care and disability compensation for veterans claiming that they were suffering from Gulf War Syndrome compared with about 50 percent of claims for other medical conditions [30]. In failing to recognize the clustering of psychogenic symptoms, historian Elaine Showalter writes that by denying the existence of "war neurosis," we do them an injustice. "The suffering of Gulf War syndrome *is* real by any measure, and symptoms caused by war neurosis are just as painful and incapacitating as those caused by chemicals, parasites or smoke. …even strong and heroic men and women, fighting a just cause, can be affected by the conversion of strong emotions into physical symptoms" [29, pp 142–143].

Stress from fear and uncertainly that accompany wars and terrorist attacks typically generate clusters of medically unexplained symptoms that have been deemed to have been of psychogenic origin. As Dr. Da Costa noted as far back as the Civil War, the appearance of a similar complex of unexplained symptoms can be found in the civilian population. For instance, after the September 11, 2001 terrorist attacks on the World Trade Center in lower Manhattan, of 10,000 New York City firefighters to visit the site of this traumatic and emotional event, about 4000 reported respiratory problems (wheezing, coughing, shortness of breath, chest pressure, and pain, general anxiety). The condition has since been labeled 'World Trade Center Syndrome.' Many others living and working near the site have exhibited similar complaints. While the number of persons affected may sound compelling, since the attacks, city, state, and federal agencies have continuously monitored the air at the site for contaminants and found them not to pose a public health problem [31, 32].

Symptoms in the American diplomats in Havana closely parallel those that are associated with war trauma – right down to the concussion-like symptoms that have often been misdiagnosed as brain trauma. In so far as the political and scientific evidence for the perpetration of an attack on US Embassy staff in Cuba is woefully inadequate – and inconclusive at best, what is the most likely scenario? That the diplomats were the target of a mysterious new weapon, sonic or otherwise, for which there is no concrete evidence, or they were suffering from psychogenic symptoms generated by the stressful situation they had found themselves in? In the case of the former explanation, for more than a century, the medical community has accumulated a vast amount of evidence for the existence of psychogenic war trauma under an array of labels: shell shock, war neuroses, combat fatigue, soldier's heart, effort syndrome, operational fatigue syndrome, and post-traumatic stress disorder. It is important to remember that each of these conditions reflect the times and manifest in slightly different forms to mirror the belief, hence, the Cuban subjects have more ear and pressure sensations, possibly reflecting the belief in a sonic attack. It is important to add that due to the large variation in symptoms, none of these conditions are truly syndromes. To this lengthy list we should add another: 'Havana Syndrome.'

References

1. Jones E, Hodgins Vermaas R, McCartney H, Everitt B, Beech C, Poynter D, et al. Post-combat syndromes from the Boer War to the Gulf War: a cluster analysis of their nature and attribution. BMJ. 2002;324:1–7.
2. Bentley S. A short history of PTSD: from Thermopylae to Hue, soldiers have always had a disturbing reaction to war. The Veteran. 2005. http://archive.vva.org/archive/TheVeteran/2005_03/feature_HistoryPTSD.htm. Accessed 10 Nov 2019.
3. Jones E, Wessely S. Shell shock to PTSD: military psychiatry from 1900 to the Gulf War. New York: Psychology Press; 2005. p. 2.

4. Da Costa J. On irritable heart: a clinical study of a form of functional cardiac disorder and its consequences. Am J Med Sci. 1871;61:17–52.
5. Jones E. Historical approaches to post-combat disorders. Philos Trans R Soc Lond Ser B Biol Sci. 2006;361:533–42. See pp. 534–7
6. Rubin R. More questions raised by concussion-like symptoms found in US diplomats who served in Havana. JAMA. 2018;319(11):1079.
7. Osborne L. Come on in, America: the United States in world war. New York: Abrams; 2017.
8. Toland E. The aftermath of battle: with the red cross in France. New York: The Macmillan Company; 1916. p. 97.
9. Alexander C. The shock of war. Smithsonian Magazine. 2010;41(5):58–64, 66. See p. 58.
10. Myers CS. A contribution to the study of shell shock. Lancet. 1915;186:316–20.
11. Myers CS. Shell shock in France 1914–1918. Cambridge: Cambridge University Press; 1940.
12. Salmon TW. The care and treatment of mental diseases and war neurosis. New York: National Committee for Mental Hygiene; 1917.
13. Loughran T. Shell shock, and the First World War: the making of a diagnosis and its histories. J Hist Med Allied Sci. 2012;67(1):94–119. https://doi.org/10.1093/jhmas/jrq052.
14. Linden S, Jones E. 'Shell shock' revisited: an examination of the case records of the national hospital in London. Med Hist. 2014;58(4):519–45. https://doi.org/10.1017/mdh.2014.51. The London Hospital was called the Hospital for the Paralyzed and Epileptic at the time
15. French and German neurologists and psychiatrists were even more barbaric. Most felt that shell shock reflected the unconscious need to escape the hell of war. Since hysterical symptoms were thought to be the product of suggestion, the soldiers had to be persuaded to abandon them. The notion that sufferers were weak-willed and even faking, was common among commanding officers, particularly generals. Heavy losses on the battlefield and the need for replacements influenced the aggressive treatments. The most common treatment used by French and German doctors was a combination of suggestion and shock therapy. German doctor Fritz Kaufman developed the "Kaufman cure" consisting of shocks and forced military drills accompanied by loudly shouted orders. Soldiers with paralysis received painful electrical impulses to the paralyzed limb until they gave up and began to move it. In Vienna, Doctors applied shocks to the mouth and testicles of soldiers with shell shock. In France, neurosurgeon Clovis Vincent organized a re-education camp along the banks of the Loire. Soldiers were shocked, threatened and abused until they gave up on their psychogenic symptoms. Vincent, who was known for his forceful personality, would do whatever it took to break a soldier's will, to the point of using extra-large electrodes to deliver a massive current. After the war, doctors on the winning side were largely forgiven for their ruthless behavior, but in Germany, some soldiers and their families sought revenge and several neurologists were chased from their offices. In Austria, psychiatrist Julius Wagner-Jauregg was charged with war crimes for his ruthless treatment of soldiers with 'shell shock' but he was eventually acquitted. Sigmund Freud was called as an expert witness at the trial. See: Scull A. Hysteria: the disturbing history. New York: Oxford University Press;2009. p. 168–73.
16. Cannon WB. Bodily changes in pain, hunger, fear and rage: an account of recent researches into the function of emotional excitement. New York: Appleton; 1915.
17. Ahrenfeldt RH. Psychiatry in the British army in the second world war. New York: Columbia University Press; 1958. p. 26.
18. Weinstein EA. Conversion disorders. In: Jones FD, Sparacino MA, Wilcox VL, Rothberg JM, Stokes JW, editors. War psychiatry. Washington, DC: Office of the Surgeon General at TMM Publications; 1995. p. 383–407.
19. Grinker RR, Spiegel JP. Men under stress. Philadelphia: Blakiston; 1945.
20. Crocq M, Crocq L. From shell shock and war neurosis to posttraumatic stress disorder: a history of psychotraumatology. Dialogues Clin Neurosci. 2000;2(1):47–55.
21. Jones E. Army psychiatry in the Korean War: the experience of 1 Commonwealth Division. Mil Med. 2000;165(4):256–60. See p. 259
22. Friedman MJ. PTSD history and overview. Washington, DC: U.S. Department of Veteran Affairs; 2016.

23. Bhattacharjee Y. Shell shock revisited: solving the puzzle of blast trauma. Science. 2008;319(5862):406–8.
24. Nelson L, Tarima S, LaRoche A, Hammeke T, Barr W, Guskiewicz K. Preinjury somatization symptoms contribute to clinical recovery after sport-related concussion. Neurology. 2016;86(20):1856–63.
25. This possibility is real given that sufferers may be in line to receive disability payments, pensions or file lawsuits which seek compensation. Symptoms may be a soldier's ticket out of a combat zone. In Germany, just before the First World War, there was an outbreak of "pension neurosis" after the government passed a law that provided pensions for victims of railway and industrial accidents who developed mental and nervous problems. With the onset of the war, the German government was determined to prevent a similar outbreak of war neurosis so they supported an unsympathetic treatment of soldiers with shell shock. Follow-up studies of people with post-concussion symptoms consistently show that those with compensation claims have more and lasting symptoms than those without compensation claims.
26. Cotton P. Veterans seeking answers to syndrome suspect they were goats in Gulf War. JAMA. 1994;271:1559–61.
27. Jaynes G. Walking wounded. Esquire. May 1994:70–6.
28. France D. The families who are dying for our country. Redbook. Sept 1994:114–7.
29. Showalter E. Hystories: hysterical epidemics and modern media. New York: Cambridge University Press; 1997.
30. Darcangelo V. VA takes tough stance on Gulf War illness. Sharon: The Herald; 2017.
31. Clauw D, Engel CC, Aronowitz R, Jones E, Kipen HM, Kroenke K, et al. Unexplained symptoms after terrorism and war: an expert consensus statement. J Occup Med. 2001;45(10):1040–8. https://doi.org/10.1097/01.jom.0000091693.43121.2f.
32. Price J. New York firefighters suffer after effects. The Washington Times. 3 Nov 2001.

Mass Hysteria Through the Ages: From St. Vitus Dance to Mystery Odors

Man is an animal suspended in webs of significance he himself has spun. I take culture to be those webs, and the analysis of it…not an experimental science in search of law but an interpretive one in search of meaning. It is explication I am after, construing social expressions on their surface enigmatical.

–Clifford Geertz [1]

Throughout history groups of people have been stricken with a curious condition for which no organic cause can be found. Twitching schoolgirls. Fainting factory workers. Collapsing marching bands. These outbreaks mirror prevailing beliefs and fears. Prior to the nineteenth century, episodes were shaped by religious beliefs and folklore and were centered around the existence of supernatural beings such as witches and demons. As a result, during the Middle Ages bouts of twitching, shaking, and demonic possession became commonplace in many parts of Europe. During modern times, outbreaks are concentrated in schools and factories, most often in response to a strange odor that is attributed to a noxious gas. Contemporary incidents reflect a preoccupation with concerns about contaminated air, food and water that arose in the West during the early 1960s with the appearance of *Silent Spring* by biologist Rachel Carson, which led to the birth of the modern environmental movement [2]. These contamination concerns have fueled many recent short-lived outbreaks that are characterized by headaches, dizziness, fainting, over-breathing, nausea, and abdominal pain.

Based on the patterning of cases, British Psychiatrist Simon Wessely has identified a subtype of mass psychogenic illness called 'anxiety hysteria' which occurs in response to the sudden exposure to an anxiety-generating stimulus. Episodes are common in developed Western countries and are lacking in pre-existing tension. They are typified by transient, benign symptoms and feature a rapid onset and recovery, with most lasting from a few hours to a day. Occasionally cases linger for weeks or months if those involved are not convinced that the perceived threat has been eliminated. Exacerbating factors include media coverage, cultural traditions, recent events, and the absence of calm, reassuring leadership.

© Springer Nature Switzerland AG 2020
R. W. Baloh, R. E. Bartholomew, *Havana Syndrome*,
https://doi.org/10.1007/978-3-030-40746-9_5

Anxiety hysteria typically reflects the imagined scenario. Shortly after the September 11, 2001 terror attacks on the United States, there were many incidents of mass psychogenic illness in response to pseudo-attacks [3]. In one case, amid fears of another terrorist incident, a deranged man riding a Maryland subway began spraying a mysterious substance at a transit authority officer. A scuffle ensued. Authorities rushed to the scene and swarmed on the man who was assumed to have been a terrorist. In the process of subduing him, the contents of the container spilled onto the ground. No less than 35 bystanders began to exhibit symptoms ranging from nausea to headaches and sore throats, believing that they had been the victims of a chemical or biological attack. The substance was later identified as a common, innocuous window cleaner [4, 5]. Another example of anxiety hysteria took place in May 2000, as a school bus in Peoria, Illinois was carrying a group of fourth-grade students on a field trip. Suddenly, one of the passengers began gulping for breath. Before long, several other passengers were gasping for air, forcing the driver to pull to the side of the road and summon emergency personnel. The first two students affected, asthmatics, had become preoccupied with their breathing after realizing they had left their inhalers at home. Seeing their distress, classmates grew anxious and began to hyperventilate. After being rushed to a nearby hospital, everyone quickly recovered [6].

Another type of mass psychogenic illness identified by Wessely occurs in an atmosphere of pre-existing tension which builds up over time. Episodes of this type are common in schools and factories in less economically developed countries, primarily in Asia and Africa. In work settings, the stimulus is usually employee dissatisfaction and poor labor-management relations, while incidents in schools are typified by strict rules and heavy workloads. Most school outbreaks of this type occur in traditional societies where male- and adult-dominated power structures foster strict disciplinary routines. Negotiation and protest channels are limited, and there is little opportunity to redress grievances. Within this repressive atmosphere, intense frustration builds-up and is internalized over weeks or months. Under the unrelenting pressure, students and workers may develop twitching, shaking, convulsions, interrupted speech, trance-like states, and spirit possession. The rarity of these outbreak types in Western factories may reflect a greater emphasis on employee rights and workplace conditions as supported by strong unions and occupational legislation, while most schools in Europe and North America have a more liberal outlook toward education and have outlawed physical punishment [7, 8].

In many non-Western countries, native healers are summoned to exorcize the 'evil spirits' that are believed to be responsible for the symptoms. While such actions often bring closure by convincing those affected that the 'demons' were real and have been chased away, in cases where the symptoms continue, outbreaks often endure for weeks or months. Such efforts occasionally backfire if they are unsuccessful as their presence lends credence to the existence of supernatural spirits, further heightening anxieties and undermining the authority of health care professionals and their claims that anxiety was the trigger. One outbreak at an all-girls' boarding school in the rural Malaysian state of Kedah during the 1980s, endured in a waxing, waning fashion for 5 years, exploding in intensity when *bomohs* (traditional Malay healers) were called in but were unsuccessful. The students were all Malay Muslims ages 13–17, and exhibited mental confusion, crying, twitching, shaking, trance states and spirit possession. The girls complained of an excessive focus on schoolwork, religious instruction and little recreation time. In the wake of media publicity over the outbreaks, the fits only subsided after an extraordinary series of events, which included a visit by former Malaysian Prime Minister Tunku Abdul Rahman, who later ordered their transfer to a more liberal school [9–16]. In August 2003, evil spirits had reportedly invaded a school in Thailand after several students experienced demonic possession and trance-like states. Buddhist monks were summoned to exorcize the 'spirits.' Over the previous 3 months, pupils at the Baan Thab Sawai School in Huai Thalaeng had been experiencing up to three 'demonic attacks' each day. A special ceremony was held to appease the ghosts, which included a letter from the provincial governor, Sunthorn Riewleung, who threatened to retaliate against the 'spirits' by destroying a spirit house at the school compound if the 'attacks' did not stop [17, 18].

Hysteria has traditionally been divided into two broad categories: motor and sensory. Motor hysteria is characterized by muscle contractions and movements such as maniacal dancing and writhing to shaking and convulsions. Sensory hysteria presents as sensory symptoms such as dizziness, headaches, nausea, and fatigue. Both can occur with mass hysteria and there can even be overlap between the two categories but overall there has been a gradual shift over time from motor hysteria to sensory hysteria, particularly in Western societies. Motor hysteria became rare in the twentieth century. An important factor in its demise is improved understanding of anatomy and physiology of the brain by both patients and physicians. Doctors have become adept at distinguishing between symptoms caused by structural brain damage and symptoms caused by psychogenic illness, such as telling the difference between epileptic seizures and hysterical convulsions. Patients recognize the bizarre nature of the motor symptoms and have gravitated toward more acceptable subjective complaints such as pain, dizziness, and fatigue. This is not to suggest that patients are willfully planning psychogenic illnesses but that the symptom complex of their illness can be a byproduct of their understanding of how the brain works and feedback they receive from their physicians. We will review the evolution from motor to sensory mass hysteria in the remainder of this chapter.

In recent years the American Psychiatric Association has dropped the use of the word 'hysteria' from their diagnostic manual, replacing it with the terms conversion disorder and functional somatic symptom disorder. This change was mainly due to the negative implications that hysteria had gained, especially from the seventeenth to the early twentieth centuries when it was used as a catch-all category for an array of medical conditions that supposedly just afflicted women. Cornell University Historian Rachael Maines writes that "Hysteria was a set of symptoms that varied greatly between individuals (and their physicians) including but not limited to fainting… congestion caused by fluid retention… nervousness, insomnia, sensations of heaviness in the abdomen, muscle spasms, shortness of breath, loss of appetite for food or for sex with the approved male partner, and sometimes a tendency to cause trouble for others." At that time the condition was thought to result from a "lack of sufficient sexual intercourse, deficiency of sexual gratification, or both" [19]. The political and social implications of a diagnosis of hysteria are obvious when one considers the role of women in these mostly male-dominated cultures. Women were second-class citizens who had to be confined and protected. They were under the control first of their father, then of their husband, and they had no political rights. The famous Greek philosopher, Aristotle, even used the susceptibility to hysteria as an explanation for why women were not fit to participate in the governing process. Blaming a wide range of symptoms and emotions on a uniquely female organ, the uterus, provided the cover to justify the view that women were inferior to males. We are well aware of these negative connotations that the word 'hysteria' has for women, but we use the term in this book for historical continuity with the stipulation that it refers to a psychophysiological (mind-body) illness that is equivalent to 'conversion disorder' and 'somatic symptom disorder' affecting both men and women.

The Middle Ages

Many medical historians believe that the earliest recorded outbreaks of mass psychogenic illness were the medieval dance manias. The origin of these bouts of motor hysteria is often attributed to stress from the impact of the Black Death (Bubonic Plague) which ravaged Europe around 1350. They point out that episodes began at a time of widespread pessimism and despair, spreading across the continent between the thirteenth and seventeenth centuries, where it was known as St. Vitus dance because participants often ended their processions in the vicinity of chapels and shrines dedicated to this saint. 'Epidemics' seized groups who engaged in intermittent, frenzied dancing which typically persisted for days or weeks. Symptoms included twitching, shaking, screaming, altered states of consciousness, demonic possession, convulsions, hyperventilation, sexually suggestive gestures, and even intercourse as some outbreaks turned into mass orgies. There was a clear ritualistic tenor to many episodes. Participants usually claimed that they were under demonic control and could not resist the urge to dance. Music was typically played during outbreaks and was considered an effective remedy. Historian Benjamin Gordon writes that: "From Italy it (the dancing mania) spread to Aachen (Aix-la Chapelle), Prussia, and one morning, without warning, the streets were filled with men and women who joined hands, formed circles and seemingly lost all control over their actions. They danced together, ceaselessly, for hours or days, and in wild delirium, the dancers collapsed and fell to the ground exhausted, groaning and sighing as if in the agonies of death." Gordon wrote that upon recuperating, "they swathed themselves tightly with cloth around their waists and resumed their convulsive movements. They contorted their bodies, writhing, screaming and jumping in a mad frenzy. One by one they fell from exhaustion, but as they fell, others of the town took their places. These wild dancers seemed insensible to external impressions." According to Gordon, dancing 'attacks' were often followed by convulsions. "The victims fell to the ground, fainting, and laboring for breath. They foamed from the mouth and suddenly sprang up to dance once again. Many later claimed that they had seen the walls of heaven split open and that Jesus and the Virgin Mary had appeared before them" [20].

Outbreaks of demonic possession among nuns in European convents became common during the late Middle Ages, fueled by strict Christian discipline in female religious orders. Young girls were often coerced into joining convents to lessen the economic burden on their families and were forced to endure a reclusive life of austerity, with vows of poverty and chastity. Nuns were often given meager diets interspersed by periods of lengthy fasting and repetitious prayer rituals, while minor transgressions of convent rules resulted in floggings. The number of outbreaks and their detailed descriptions in European history books is extraordinary. One case alone involving a convent of nuns in Loudun, France between 1632 and 1634, has resulted in the publication of no less than 100 books. Father Urban Grandier was blamed for bewitching the nuns and was burned at the stake [21]. During this period it was widely believed that humans could be possessed by certain animals. Wolves, sheep, cows, and dogs were widely believed to have served as familiars with the Devil, assisting them in their nefarious activities. In France, cats were particularly despised. Historian Robert Darnton writes that in parts of France, cats were so loathed that "they burned a dozen cats at a time in a basket on top of a bonfire... [while] Parisians liked to incinerate cats by the sackful" [22].

Beliefs about animals and demons helped to color the content of the trance and possession states of the nuns during this period. Hence, there are numerous cases of nuns being stricken by convulsions and behaving like animals [23]. In 1491 at Cambrai, France, a group of Sisters scampered through the fields barking like dogs [24]. At Xante, Spain in 1690, nuns "bleated like sheep, tore off their veils, [and] had convulsions in church" [25, p 393]. At a French convent, they would meow like cats for hours each day. German physician Justus Friedrich Hecker writes: "I have read in a good medical work that a nun, in a very large convent in France, began to meow like a cat; shortly afterwards other nuns also meowed. At last all the nuns meowed together every day at a certain time for several hours together. The whole surrounding Christian neighborhood heard, with equal chagrin and astonishment, this daily cat-concert, which did not cease until all the nuns were informed that a company of soldiers were placed by the police before the entrance of the convent, and that they were provided with rods, and would continue whipping them until they promised not to meow any more" [26, p 127].

An outbreak of 'hysterics' among a group of nuns at the Franciscan convent of Sainte Brigitte near Lille, in northern France, involved fantastic claims and confessions, with symptoms enduring from 1608 to 1618. When several nuns accused Sister Marie de Sains of causing their fits of demonic possession, Sister Marie gave a detailed account of the witches' Sabbath. Witchcraft historian Rosemary Guiley summarizes these activities: "The witches copulated with devils and each other in a natural fashion Mondays and Tuesdays, practiced sodomy on Thursday, and bestiality on Saturdays and sang litanies to the Devil on Wednesdays and Fridays" [27]. As is typical of convent outbreaks, under the pressure of her inquisitors, Sister Marie broke down and admitted to being in cahoots with Satan against the children of

Lille. She confessed to having disemboweled living children and killing numerous others as a sacrifice to the Devil. She claimed that after strangling them, she crushed their still-beating hearts. For her perceived crimes, Sister Marie was imprisoned for life, despite the physical impossibility of having committed many of the acts she had claimed. As part of her confession, she asserted: "I have cut the throats of a great many children in this town and in the neighbourhood, and when they were put in the ground, I dug them up and took them to our nocturnal assemblies. I killed a lot of them thus, or else I poisoned them with poison given me by the demons. Sometimes I pulled their hair out, or pierced their hearts or temples with needles." Despite her incredible claims and clear indications that she was mentally deranged, influenced by the beliefs of the times, she received little sympathy. She further claimed to "have thrown many [children] into flaming furnaces; I have drowned others; I have roasted many on a spit; I have boiled others in pots or threw them into the latrines; some I burnt alive, others I gave to lions to eat, or wolves, serpents and other animals; I have hung some up by their legs, arms or necks, or by their shame-ful parts; I have smashed their heads against the wall, then I have flayed them and cut them into pieces as though to salt them. Others I threw to the dogs. There are some that I crucified, to insult the Saviour…" [28].

One remarkable series of outbreaks occurred at the Louviers nunnery in Normandy, France, between 1642 and 1647, after a group of nuns were stricken with bouts of twitching, convulsions and demonic possession. The malady appeared after they were forced to worship in the nude. The nuns were also under extreme duress. In order to show their worthiness and gain divine favor, one historian observes that they engaged in a variety of self-torments including "passing their nights in prayer, fasting with excessive strictness, torturing their flesh with flagellation, and to crown all these fine works, rolling half-naked in the snow" [29, p 73]. The roots of the outbreak can be traced back to the opening of the convent in 1616 and its chaplain, Father Pierre David, as an Adamite believed that people should worship in a natural state to show humility before god just as Adam and Eve had presumably done. As a result, Father David ordered the nuns to strip naked during communion services. This situation created extraordinary sexual tension, conflict and guilt as the nuns began to have liaisons with their fellow sisters and priests. In her autobiography, Sister Bavente writes of some of what then transpired: "The most holy, virtuous, and faithful nuns were held to be those who stripped themselves completely naked and danced before him in that state, appeared naked in choir, and sauntered naked through the gardens. Nor was that all" [25, p 320]. After the nude worship and the resulting sexual shena-nighans had gained the attention of church authorities, an investigation was con-ducted in 1643. The two senior priests at the convent were convicted of conspiring with the devil and burned alive. Church officials were especially harsh in their criti-cism of Father Picard for his role in initiating the affair, but they could not punish him as he had died a year earlier. They were so incensed that they ordered his body dug up and burned. As for the fate of the nuns, they were viewed as the victims of bewitch-ment and were dispersed to other convents [25, pp 319–23].

One of the last nunnery outbreaks took place between 1745 and 1749 when an outburst of 'hysterics' struck six nuns at a convent in Unterzell, Germany. Those affected exhibited demonic possession, entered trance-like states, foamed at the mouth and suffered from bouts of "suffocation." On several occasions, the nuns would disrupt mass by crying out and exhibiting an array of sexually explicit gestures and contort their bodies in sexually suggestive ways. Soon Maria Renata von Mossau was publicly accused by a dying nun that she had bewitched her and the others. After being tortured and confessing to fantastic tales, Maria was beheaded before a cheering crowd, her body tossed into a bonfire [25, pp 408–14].

Outbreaks involving people who were seemingly possessed by animals were not confined to convents; similar episodes occurred at schools and orphanages during the sixteenth and seventeenth centuries. In 1566, about 30 children at an orphanage in Amsterdam, Holland, were afflicted with violent spasms. At times the children entered trance-like states and behaved like cats, climbing across rooftops on all fours [30, p 17, 31, p 521]. In 1673, children at an orphanage in Hoorn, Holland, began to scream, shout and bark like dogs. The trigger for these and kindred episodes was religious discipline in response to the fear of witchcraft. Dutch pastor Balthasar Bekker who was an influential figure in ending the witchcraft persecutions of early modern Europe was a witness to the events. "They tugged and tore at themselves, striking at the ground with their legs and arms and even with their heads, crying, yelling and barking like dogs so that it was a terrifying thing to see." He wrote that some of their bellies "pounded so fearfully, that one would have said there was a living creature moving about inside them or even that a barrel was being rolled within their bodies. So strong were these movements that it took three, four, five or even six persons to hold them: one would take the head, two others the hands, one sat on the legs and sometimes another to sit on the belly to prevent them moving" [30, p 517]. Eventually, the spasms would subside and those affected would lie motionless, their bodies as "stiff as a bar of iron, so that with one person holding the head and another the feet, they could be carried anywhere, without making any movement. Sometimes this happened for several hours on end, and even at night, until 11 pm, midnight, one, two or three o'clock." The fits seem to have been prompted by a strict regime of religious instruction and prayer. In an attempt to stop the outbreak, they were forced to endure even lengthier prayer sessions, but this had the opposite effect, intensifying their symptoms [30].

Saint-Médard Pilgrim Outbreak

Mass psychogenic illness has taken many forms through the ages. In France during the 1730s, followers of the writings of Cornelius Jansen (1585–1638) flocked to the Saint-*Médard* cemetery and the grave of a pious deacon, after reports spread that the site had been the scene of miracles. Soon people from all over Paris arrived to participate in emotionally charged worship, which included outbreaks of mass spirit possession. The stage for this episode was set in 1727 with the burial of François de Paris, who's views were considered heretical by the Catholic Church. Many people considered him a saint due to his work with the poor and downtrodden. One day, a woman was paying her respects to her fallen hero at his tomb in the cemetery, when she reported being cured. Soon others visited the tomb and claimed to have been miraculously healed [32].

During the public outbursts, one observer said that the entire square at the cemetery and nearby streets "were full of girls, women, ill people of all ages, convulsing as if in competition of one with another. Here were men falling to the ground like real epileptics, while ... others, a bit further on, swallow pebbles, [and] glass fragments ..." [33, p 75]. The spectacle was remarkable as some women stretched out their bodies on the ground and begged spectators to strike them or for people to sit on them. They said these actions gave them relief. A consensus was soon reached by worshipers, that in order to be cured, one first had to experience the convulsions and related symptoms. It soon became fashionable for people to visit the cemetery for the sole purpose of watching the wild scenes. In January 1732, worried over their growing popularity and the threat they posed to public order, King Louis XV ordered the cemetery closed. Instead of causing the movement to die down, it went underground and was practiced in the cellars and attics of private homes. Historian Richard Madden writes that the phenomena exhibited by the convulsionnaires included "ecstasies, raptures, insensibility to pain, rigidity of muscles, submission of the will and the senses to the volition of another person... Increased... quickness of perception, heightened powers of imagination, a vivid energising influence, fraught with enthusiasm and even eloquence; claims to clairvoyance..." [23, p 541].

A prominent supporter of the movement was Louis Carrè de Montgeron, an advisor to the Parliament. In 1737, he was thus imprisoned, where he died in 1754. He recalls how he provided relief for one particular convulsionnaire, 23-year-old Jeanne Moler, who leaned against a wall while he struck her in the stomach with a firedog – metal supports used to hold logs in fireplaces. The account, while dramatic and graphic, was not untypical, as convulsionnaires claimed that being physically assaulted helped to cure them. He wrote:

> I began by giving relatively light blows. However, excited by her complaints which left me in no doubt that she wanted harder blows, I redoubled my efforts; but in vain I employed all my strength. She continued to complain that the blows I was giving her were so feeble, that they didn't give her any solace, and she made me hand the iron to a stronger man. Having watched me, he realised that no blows that he could give her would be too violent, he discharged terrible blows, always in the pit of the stomach. The girl received 100 from him, over and above the 60 I had given her which she found so feeble. Only then did she cry out with joy which was reflected on her face and in her eyes: Ha! that's so good! ah, that does me such good! Take heart, my brother, double the force, if you can [32, p 692].

Observers looked on in amazement as followers went into violent spasms, thrashing on the ground near the gravestones oblivious of their surroundings. Touching the tomb was enough to provoke the convulsions: and indeed, it was not necessary for the sufferer to actually visit the cemetery, for sachets of soil from the ground near the tomb, taken to them, would do the trick. In January 1732, the authorities, ostensibly in the interest of public order but also concerned that the Jansenists were winning too much sympathy, closed the cemetery, provoking a famous graffito: *By the king's command, no miracle may be performed in this place.* For a while, the faithful got around this by waiting for a burial to take place, then crowding in along with the coffin. Soon authorities banned all burials in the cemetery. The effect did not deter the convulsionnaires, it simply drove them elsewhere. Everyday life was so disrupted by the daily pandemonium, that in 1732 the King ordered the cemetery closed and forbade convulsing publicly. This only strengthened the movement as people met across Paris in private homes. The King next proclaimed by decree that anyone caught convulsing in hysterics would be jailed. This slowed but did not extinguish the movement [33, p 75], which continued in a clandestine fashion for much of the century.

The Modern Era of Secular Outbreaks

During the nineteenth century, many European schools were the scene of twitching, convulsions, and trance states. The affected schools shared several common elements: they were among the strictest in their rules, regulations and educational rigor. Episodes coincided with the rise of the educational fad of "mental discipline," which held that the mind could be trained like a muscle through repetition. A teaching method developed in the writings of the German philosopher Christian von Wolff in 1734, and popularized in the latter part of the century by Scottish writer Thomas Reid, this new approach to learning was widely accepted throughout much of Europe during the latter half of the century before rapidly losing popularity by the beginning of World War I. Some administrators took this method to extreme levels. Students were under pressure to perform in a curriculum that was repetitive such as monotonous drills in memorization, writing, and arithmetic. There was little in the way of spontaneity, creativity or individuality. According to the results of a 1908 British inquiry on the European education system, some German school districts were so strict that even "corporal punishment in the elementary schools is harsh and severe," [34, p 215] with some schools instilling discipline that resembled what one might find in the German military, including rigid obedience, an obsession with order, uniformity and self-control [35]. School inspector Joseph Lucas wrote in 1878 that in Bavaria, "it truly does not matter if one serves his 3 years in the army or in the schoolhouse" [36, p 475]. One German curriculum issued to elementary school teachers in 1890, was typical for its uncompromising rigidity: "In order to save time, maintain order and quiet, and accustom the children to uniform activity and to 'obedience and command,' it is recommended that every activity which occurs daily or which is frequently repeated be regulated by orders and done in time" [37]. Indeed, in 1895, the *Frankischer Kurier* newspaper estimated that over the course of the first 6 years in school, the typical student had memorized 1258 lines, 26 hymns, and 350 sayings. It was within this backdrop of tedious, repetitive drills in memorizing, mental arithmetic, and handwriting, that strange symptoms appeared. In 1893, girls at the People's School in Valle, Austria, were stricken with convulsions and seizures. Students would complain of dizziness and a buzzing in the ears before passing out, after which their bodies would heave and convulse, and they would foam at the mouth [38, p 231]. The previous year a peculiar contagion affected a Catholic girls' school in a region of Germany notorious for its strict schooling. A group of girls fell into a strange daze and "could not be awakened by shaking, calling or even by pricking with pins." Some of the girls went into violent convulsions [39].

Between June and September 1892, a writing tremor struck 20 pupils at a village school in Gross-tinz, Germany [40]. The episode began on June 28 when a 10-year-old girl suddenly began trembling in her right hand. Soon her entire body was shaking. After half an hour, the trembling subsided, and she was fine for the rest of the day. The next day several other girls in the same class began to exhibit hand tremors lasting from 30 minutes to an hour. With each passing day the trembling lasted longer and longer. Soon tremors were affecting their entire bodies and making it impossible for the girls to complete their writing assignments. At this point, with each new case, the girls, as young as 5 and as old as 12, were immediately removed from the classroom in hopes of stemming the tide. New cases of tremor soon appeared in previously healthy girls. Between July 14 and 20, the symptoms peaked. "On almost every seat were patients having convulsions of the whole body. The girls fell under the seats and had to be carried from the room by the boys" [38, p 233]. At this point, 20 of the school's 38 girls were affected, 8 of whom had lost consciousness during the attacks. The 'fits' would last from between 15 minutes to an hour and subside gradually. Those exhibiting signs of unconsciousness, upon awakening, said they "knew absolutely nothing of what had happened" [38, p 229]. On July 20 administrators took drastic steps. The crisis growing worse by the day, they sent all the girls home but had the school's 32 boys attend classes for the next week, at which point all students were dismissed for summer vacation. The school reopened on August 19. Upon resumption of classes, the trembling and convulsions ceased, though administrators had a new problem – several girls were now reporting incapacitating headaches and were sent home to recuperate. The drama finally ended after the Autumn [38].

An 1893 outbreak occurred at a girl's school in southern Germany. The investigating physician described a procession of weeping girls, making wild, exaggerated gestures. At times they would break into bouts of uncontrollable laughing. He observed: "They were in groups of two or three, in each of which one was led by another or dragged along by two. Those who were dragged usually hung unconscious in the arms of their companions, head sunk upon the breast, and the legs dragging upon the floor." Several other girls were unconscious, and still others were sighing convulsively and crying. Their schoolmates looked on in amazement [41]. Between 1905 and 1906, a 'trembling disease' swept through several schools in Meissen, Germany, the symptoms afflicting otherwise healthy children who had excessive writing assignments. The episode began in October 1905 when the hands of a 13-year-old girl began to twitch and shake. Gradually more cases appeared. By the time students returned from Christmas break the trembling continued to escalate through February 21, at which point 134 students had been affected. Administrators then closed the school until March 14, but it failed to stem the tide and over the next 3 weeks 237 students were stricken. But then, presumably with all of the time off from writing, the pent-up tension slowly dissipated, and the episode seems to have ended in mid-May [38]. According to the German journal *Muenchener Medizinsche Wochenschrift,* those who 'caught' the 'disease' were 9- to 13-year-old girls from the elementary and middle schools [42].

The Power of Belief

Attempts to focus on character traits of the victims of mass psychogenic illness by asking the question, 'Why do some workers or students fall ill, while their colleagues do not,' have met with a dead end. There is no 'mass hysteria'-prone personality. While some victims have scored higher on scales for neuroticism [43, 44], paranoia [45], and hysterical traits [46], others have not [47–51]. A study in the United States found an association between student grades and their likelihood of being stricken [52], while a similar study in Singapore found no link [53]. Some researchers observed that those affected had low intelligence quotients [54], yet other studies drew the opposite conclusion [47, 55]. What is clear from this research is the importance of focusing on the beliefs of those affected and to view episodes through the eyes of the participants. Just as people get caught up in watching a movie and temporarily suspend their judgment, once people 'buy into' a belief which is often supported by friends and relatives, the power of the nocebo effect can take over as people who think they are unwell, might begin to feel unwell. British psychiatrist David Taylor supports this view: "In these dramas the actors and the audience are equal partners. When the sick are presented to doctors the doctors are compelled to act from their perspective just as the parents or the crowd acted from theirs. In this way, the medical procedures tend to validate the sickness to the relatives in the same process which invalidates it to the doctors" [56, p 395]. Of vital importance, Taylor writes, is the context of the outbreak. "Epidemic hysterias arise couched in social settings that enhance emotionality and promote the rapid 'mental acceptance of propositions as true even if beyond observations.' The sorts of events that produce these responses are unavoidable apparent threats that have emerged through some form of ultra-rapid group consensus" [56, p 395]. This perspective is consistent with the notion that most victims of psychogenic outbreaks are normal, healthy people who are exhibiting a collective stress response. Through an accident of history and circumstance, they become part of the same drama, which through the nocebo effect, became real in its consequences.

Anthropologist Clifford Geertz once wrote that understanding human behavior was "not an experimental science in search of law but an interpretative one in search of meaning" [1, p 5]. Instead of looking at the seemingly bizarre nature of the symptoms or abnormalities in the actors involved, we need to focus on the drama itself. This was evident in one of the first recorded outbreaks of mass psychogenic illness in a British cotton factory in Lancashire. It was investigated by a Dr. W. St. Clare who wrote that:

> ...a girl, on the fifteenth of February, 1787, put a mouse into the bosom of another girl, who had a great dread of mice. The girl was immediately thrown into a fit, and continued in it with

the most violent convulsions, for 24 hours. On the following day, three more girls were seized in the same manner; and on the 17th, six more. By this time the alarm was so great, that the whole work, in which 200 or 300 were employed, was totally stopped, and an idea prevailed that a particular disease had been introduced by a bag of cotton opened in the house. ...Dr St. Clare was sent for from Preston; before he arrived three more were seized, and during that night and the morning of the 19th, eleven more, making in all twenty-four. Of these, twenty-one were young women, two were girls of about ten years of age, and one man, who had been much fatigued with holding the girls... The symptoms were anxiety, strangulation, and very strong convulsions; and these were so violent as to last without any intermission from a quarter of an hour to twenty-four hours, and to require four or five persons to prevent the patients from tearing their hair and dashing their heads against the floor or walls.

The symptoms soon subsided [57].

It is important to understand that outbreaks of mass psychogenic illness change with the times to reflect prevailing beliefs. A key element is plausibility. It is with this insight that the events in Cuba and among diplomatic staff in places like China and Uzbekistan, are best understood. The stage for the 'sonic attack' saga had been set decades earlier during the Cold War. Harassment and surveillance of American personnel was not only well-known, it was expected. Within this foreign, hostile work environment, Embassy staff began to redefine the mundane sounds of mating insects and vague illness symptoms, as being caused by nefarious agents from Cuba or their allies.

The Power of an Idea: 'Fried' Mail and 'Bad' Coke

Contemporary cases of mass psychogenic illness are dominated by contamination fears involving strange odors and scenarios about imaginary terrorists. The appearance of cases in this category exploded after the September 11 terror attacks on America. In the wake of the anthrax mail attacks attributed to possible terrorists during the fall of 2001, the US Postal Service began processing mail by passing it through irradiation machines where letters and packages are bombarded with radiation designed to kill biological agents such as anthrax. Soon after the devices began operating, postal workers handling the treated mail began to exhibit mysterious symptoms including nausea, headaches, eye irritation, skin rashes, and a metallic taste. Congress quickly launched an investigation.

In a commentary in the *Bulletin of the Atomic Scientists,* Bret Lortie was critical of the probe, viewing it as a waste of time and taxpayer money. While it may appear arrogant for scientists to dismiss these health issues without any further investigation, he pointed out that the science behind irradiation was sound and had already been the subject of numerous studies – all proving it to be safe. He wrote: "As any reader of the *Bulletin* knows, irradiating mail is akin to microwaving it: There's no residual radiation. Unfortunately Sen. Charles Grassley didn't know that before requesting a full investigation" [58]. One of the firms tasked with carrying out the irradiation, Titan Scan Technologies of Lima, Ohio, issued a statement through their spokesman Wil Williams. "It just doesn't make sense ... Either they're getting sick from something else or it's mass hysteria," he said. Williams noted that while new to postal workers, irradiation had been used for years in the medical profession, without problems. "When medical people open up cartons of supplies that have been irradiated, they don't get sick. After a decade of using this process worldwide, all of a sudden somebody [in Washington] is saying there are health consequences" [59, 60].

In response to the perceived crisis, the US Office of Compliance distributed 14,000 surveys to workers in the House and Senate, asking if they had any health problems linked to handling mail. Of the meager 215 workers who replied, the prevalence of symptoms involved headaches, rashes, itchiness, nausea, burning eyes, and bloody noses – all common in the general population. Despite the survey, Congress ordered the National Institute for Occupational Safety and Health (NIOSH) to analyze air at the Capitol for "contaminants that could be on the irradiated mail – such as carbon monoxide, volatile organic compounds, formaldehyde, ozone, polynuclear aromatic hydrocarbons, toluene, and particulate matter…" The levels were either below those that could impair health or zero [58].

In January 2002, 11 workers for the US Commerce Department in Washington DC, developed breathing difficulties, throat irritation and nausea after handling irradiated mail. An inspection found the building to be free of hazardous materials, leading federal law enforcement officials to conclude that the cause was "mass hysteria." While some employees were worried that the large number of letters with plastic wrapping or plastic address windows would emit hazardous fumes when irradiated, government officials were adamant that irradiated mail does not emit toxic fumes. One possible factor contributing to the outbreak is the number of urban legends about irradiation [59, 60]. After conducting their investigation into the health concerns of the postal workers, the NIOSH concluded that the complaints by mail handlers were psychological in origin [58].

The Belgian Coca-Cola Scare

On the afternoon of June 8, 1999, 10 children from a Catholic secondary school in the town of Bornem, near Antwerp in Belgium became sick [61]. Since there was no doctor on staff they were taken to a nearby hospital as the school nurse and other staff frantically tried to identify a possible cause. The only explanation that they could find was that all of the sick children had consumed containers of Coca-Cola at lunch. When questioned, the girls reported that the Coke had an abnormal odor and taste but the description of the odor varied from child to child. The staff then went from classroom to classroom asking students if they had drunk Coca-Cola at lunch and if they felt sick [62]. This prompted a second wave of students to fall ill and were taken to the hospital, followed by a third group who were taken in the evening when they were stricken after returning home from school. The main symptoms were headaches, dizziness, nausea, difficulty catching breath, malaise, abdominal discomfort and trembling. Blood and urine samples were normal. Of the 33 children taken to the hospital, 18 were released and 15 remained overnight for further observation. Four more students were admitted the next morning with identical symptoms, bringing the total number affected to 37. Just over three times the number of girls were affected than boys [63].

The Bornem incident received massive publicity in the Belgian media that night and by the following week throughout Europe. The idea that Coca-Cola was poisoning children was front-page news. The context of the outbreak contributed to the tension surrounding it, including a lack of government confidence. Belgians were just recovering from what was dubbed "the dioxin crisis" earlier in the year after a tank filled with recycled fats used in the production of animal feed was accidentally contaminated with dioxin and other pollutants. Hundreds of Belgian farmers fed the tainted feed to their animals, triggering widespread fears that consuming the affected animal products could harm their health. In May 1999, the media reported that chickens had been contaminated with dioxin, causing widespread anxiety. Chickens and eggs were recalled followed by dairy and meat products. For a while, people were afraid to eat *any* meat products. Making matters worse, while the contamination occurred in February, it was not made public until May 25 when news of the incident was leaked to the press. The uproar eroded government trust and resulted in the forced resignations of the Ministers for Health and Agriculture just prior to the June elections. The media questioned the safety of modern-day foods and scientists emphasized that even minuscule amounts of chemicals could seriously affect health. The dioxin scare was on everyone's mind and was a major topic of conversation in the media in most homes when the tainted Coke scare struck.

After the Bornem outbreak on June 8, outbreaks of similar symptoms attributed to drinking Coke or other Coca-Cola products occurred at four other schools in northern Belgium in rapid succession, first in the scenic city of Brugge on June 10, followed by Harelbeke on June 11, and finally the cities of Kortrijk and Lochriste on June 14. A total of 75 children, mostly girls, were affected at the four schools. Most drank Coca-Cola or Fanta from cans produced at a different plant than the bottled Coke responsible for the Bornem outbreak. The outbreak soon spread to the general population as large numbers of adults reported that they too became sick after drinking Coke and other soft drinks made by the company. The Belgium Poison Control Center was flooded with phone calls from citizens all over the country. Of 1418 calls received between June 8 and 20 in relation to the consumption of soft drinks, 943 reported becoming ill after drinking Coke, and to a lesser degree other soft drinks, even some made by other companies. The number of calls peaked on June 15· and rapidly declined [64].

Overwhelmed with the reaction in Belgium, the Coca-Cola conglomerate did what companies are generally expected to do in such circumstances: they accepted responsibility and apologized. They even took out full-page ads in local newspapers and CEO Douglas Ivester hinted that there may have been a problem at the bottling plant in Antwerp. They announced a recall of Coke and Fanta bottles and cans with certain code numbers on June 11, but on June 14 the newly appointed Health Minister banned the sale of all Coca-Cola products in Belgium. He wanted to dramatically show his concern for public health and his willingness to take on potent economic interests, traits that his predecessor was accused of lacking. The ban on Coca-Cola products was estimated to cost the company between 100 and 250 million dollars [65]. Soon all Coca-Cola products were ordered off the shelves in

France, Spain, Germany, Holland, and Luxembourg. Similar symptoms were reported in France after residents consumed soft drinks, and to a lesser degree in other European countries but these outbreaks were not documented.

Was Coca-Cola responsible for the Belgium outbreaks? An internal investigation by the company identified two separate potential sources of contamination: one at the bottling plant and the other at the canning facility [62]. The Bornem outbreak could have been caused by contamination of the carbon dioxide (CO_2) with carbonyl sulfide (COS) which can hydrolyse to foul smelling hydrogen sulfide (H_2S). Company officials suggested that there may have been a problem with the carbonation process since they found tiny amounts of foul-smelling H_2S in some of the bottles. At the canning plant they also found traces of 4-chloro-3-methylphenol on the outside of some cans, probably from the application of a fungicide on the wooden pallets used for transportation. Like hydrogen sulfide, this compound also has a distinct odor. When these findings were reviewed by independent toxicologists, they concluded that the chemicals were in such small quantities, they could not have caused the illnesses even though they might have produced an odor. A panel of experts organized by the Belgian Health Ministry came to a similar conclusion and further reported that no other notable chemical toxins had been found despite extensive studies. Their verdict was mass hysteria. They suggested that the outbreak was triggered by odors associated with trace amounts of chemicals and occurred in a population stressed by the dioxin scare. Despite a large number of children and adults with minor symptoms, not a single subject had a life-threatening condition. They emphasized that clinical and laboratory tests in the children and adults and the geographical spread of the outbreak were not consistent with a toxic or infectious agent. This startling conclusion was presented to the public in a television program on June 23 and presented to the scientific community in a letter to the English journal *The Lancet* on July 3, 1999 [66]. There was an immediate backlash from physicians and the public who questioned the panel's assessment. They were accused of drawing their conclusion "without having seen a single patient" or of "being wise after the fact." They countered by noting that sometimes it is better to be able to stand back and examine all of the facts at a distance. As time went on and no further cases were identified, the public began to accept the mass hysteria diagnosis. The ban on Coca-Cola products in Belgium was lifted on June 23 but the Belgium government did not officially accept the psychogenic illness hypothesis until March 31 of the following year.

In retrospect, the Coca-Cola company appears to have contributed to the spread of illness to other schools and the general public by immediately taking responsibility without concrete evidence that their product was dangerous. This increased the public's concern about the safety of Coke products. The company was in a no-win situation. If they delayed responding or denied culpability, they ran the risk of being accused of a cover-up. Suggesting the possibility of psychogenic illness early on when children were becoming sick, could have been a public relations disaster. The company's insistence in holding onto their "secret formula" for the production of Coca-Cola certainly hindered the investigation. Toxicologists needed to know the steps in the production of Coke in order to assess the company's data and to perform their own analyses. They complained that the company had sent them scant documentation. Belgium's Deputy Prime Minister even suggested that "the corporation deserved the recall and bad press for not being more forthcoming" [62].

As with most cases of mass psychogenic illness, medical personnel and the media play an important role in the event. The media reinforced anxiety and public anger. They made frequent comparisons between the dioxin and Coca-Cola crises in headlines and editorials and showed pictures of loads of dead animals being dumped alongside crates of soft drinks being disposed of. First responders and emergency room physicians were obviously concerned in the face of a possible mass poisoning incident, especially in children and appropriately took the matter seriously. The media picked up on these concerns and reported the Coca-Cola poisoning as fact. But as it became obvious that none of the children were seriously ill and most were recovering quickly with no untoward effects, reassurance was appropriate for both the children and their families. Physicians at the Poison Control Center were obviously convinced of a poisoning epidemic and may have unwittingly contributed to the spread by directing all callers to go to their physician or to a hospital [61]. The Center identified other potential incidents. On June 11, a physician called the Poison Control Center to ask if there had been any reports of hemolysis from drinking Coca-Cola. Hemolysis is a rupture of red blood cells that can be a sign of serious poisoning. This prompted the staff to record hemolysis as a possible effect of drinking Coke and the Health Minister picked up on this and mentioned it at a press conference. Not long after, a hospital reported 10 cases of hemolysis after consumption of Coke, which was immediately broadcast by the media. While the 'smoking gun' of the 'poisoning' had seemingly been identified, a team of hematologists, found *no evidence for hemolysis* and concluded that the report was due to a technical artifact.

Recurrent Themes

A more recent example of the power of belief to trigger physical symptoms occurred on September 21, 2018, when upwards of 50 students at a New Zealand middle school began to feel unwell shortly after a plane flew low over the building. In the current international political climate and amid news reports about terrorist incidents in Europe and the United States, some of the students surmised that the plane had dropped poison. The plane's appearance coincided with the presence of a strong ammonia and sulphur-like smell. One of the students claimed to have seen a "white substance" fall from the plane. Symptoms included headaches, skin irritation, and vomiting [67]. Ten pupils were taken to hospital for assessment; all were discharged a short time later [68]. An investigation revealed that the smell had resulted from a pile of steaming compost that had been dumped near the school at the same time the plane flew over [69]. Outbreaks of psychogenic illness result from a confluence of events that often appear to be unique, yet it is remarkable how similar episodes recur. For instance, on April 22, 1936, a mysterious illness spread through the East Highland Grammar School in Columbus, Georgia, affecting 19 students and a teacher. The symptoms appeared at the same time a low-flying plane had passed over the school, leading to the belief that the building had been drenched in toxic chemicals. The incident happened at a time when there was much media reporting about the possible use of chemical weapons in warfare. As in the New Zealand incident, authorities determined that the plane's appearance was unrelated to the illness cluster [70].

Strange odors and contamination rumors are a recurring contemporary theme. An example of an odor scare occurred at Warren County High School in McMinnville, Tennessee on November 12, 1998. Shortly after arriving to work, a teacher developed a headache, dizziness, nausea and had difficulty catching her breath after she thought that she smelled gasoline in her classroom [71]. Several students in the same room began to develop similar symptoms. The teacher set off a fire alarm to evacuate the school, during which many other students also began developing similar symptoms as they observed the dramatic arrival of firefighters, police and first responders. The teacher and several students were rushed to the hospital. By the end of that day, 80 students, 19 staff, and 1 family member who came to pick up a child, were taken to the local emergency room reporting symptoms they believed were caused by something in the school; 38 were kept overnight for observation. After a detailed investigation over the next 2 days by the fire department, the gas company and the Occupational Safety and Health Administration (OSHA), no toxic source was found, and the school was reopened amid fears that a toxin was the cause but had not been found. The next morning on November 17, more students fell sick, ambulances were called, and 71 more pupils were taken to the hospital. The school was again closed, and the principal contacted several government agencies to conduct an even more thorough investigation in the search for a toxic trigger.

What followed was a massive response coordinated by the Environmental Protection Agency (EPA), with help from the Agency for Toxic Substances and Disease Registry, OSHA, The Tennessee Department of Health, The Tennessee Department of Agriculture, private contractors and local emergency officials. The air was surveyed to identify potential contaminants. The school's air handling, plumbing, and structural systems were examined. Authorities left no stone unturned, going so far as to check local caves and sample groundwater. A nearby spring and river were also examined for a wide range of chemicals. No abnormalities were found on any of these samples and the laboratory tests performed on victims were also negative. Public announcements that the school was safe and that the tests were negative were widely broadcast but no mention was made of mass psychogenic illness. Health officials were reluctant to issue a public statement due to the stigma and anger that such diagnoses tend to elicit. Interestingly, three senior officials in the state health department independently suggested mass psychogenic illness as the probable cause early on but due to the intense anxiety in the community, they felt obligated to pursue the investigation beyond what they considered necessary. The press played a role in stoking fears. Local media coverage was intense and even more than a month after the outbreak, it continued to report on people with persistent symptoms believed to be due to toxic exposure at the school, rumors of a government coverup, and incompetence in handling the case. Many people remained certain that a mysterious toxin caused the illness, but it had not been found. Some even suggested that the massive investigation itself proved that a toxin *had* been found but was covered up.

Ninety-nine patients responded to an open-ended question about what they thought caused their illness. Two-thirds believed it was fumes or some other toxic substance. One hundred and twenty or 65 percent reported smelling an unusual odor before becoming sick. Remarkably, they used 30 different words to describe the smell in 31 different locations throughout the school. One month after the outbreak, a sample of 284 students who had been present in classrooms at the time, completed a questionnaire. Twenty-five percent reported symptoms during the outbreak. Those with the illness were significantly more likely to have observed another person fall ill during the episode, knew a classmate who was ill or smelled an odor at the school, compared with those without the illness.

Costs associated with the outbreak were substantial [71]. Medical expenses for the emergency room and hospital visits alone were estimated at $100,000. Testing for toxins required more than 200 work-hours and at least $14,000 for lab supplies and more than 3000 person-hours were spent by personnel from 12 government agencies, 8 laboratories, and 7 private consulting groups. The estimated total was well into the millions of dollars without considering the costs of the disruption to the community.

Sometimes episodes involving contamination fears are better managed in developing countries than in the United States because they have less government and community resources to spend on the outbreaks and there is often less media coverage of the events. However, these countries still have to deal with concerned parents and community leaders and with social and mass media. A recent report of an outbreak of mass psychogenic illness in an all-girls school in Bangladesh illustrates these points. On April 14, 2013, five students in a girl's high school in Gopalganj, Bangladesh reported feeling sick within a few minutes after morning tiffin (a snack or light breakfast) [72]. As news of the sickness spread through the school, several more students became ill and were taken to the emergency department of a nearby hospital. Many students who helped transport the sick girls to the hospital also became ill. Most of the sick girls reported that the cake they were fed had a bad odor or taste. The 93 students who were admitted to the hospital underwent routine tests and then received reassurance and counseling. There was a wide range of symptoms: abdominal pain (83 percent), headache (73 percent), general body ache (63 percent), weakness and fatigue (61 percent), chest pain (69 percent), a burning sensation (54 percent) and dizziness (42 percent). The situation was stabilizing until the media and anxious parents began arriving at the hospital and the police were called to help manage the crowds. Reports of a mysterious illness were broadcast on all the major television networks and rumors of a few deaths rapidly spread through the community. Political leaders and curious locals descended on the hospital. The situation was gradually controlled as doctors, nurses and hospital officials reassured the students and their parents that no serious problem existed. By now, many of the students had recovered enough to be discharged that evening and nearly all were sent home within 2 days. Seventeen were briefly re-hospitalized. The parents of three students were not reassured by the statements from hospital officials, so they took their children to see specialists. The suspicious cake was sent for microbiological and toxicological testing. The results were unremarkable.

A detailed questionnaire was given to all students who were admitted to the hospital. Ninety-eight percent of the sick girls reported having eaten the suspect cake, of these, 88 percent noticed an unpleasant smell or taste. Sixty-three percent reported first becoming sick while helping to transport other sick girls to the hospital, and 20 percent after seeing other sick girls in the school. Finally, 11 percent became sick after watching TV reports of the event at home. Most of the girls were ages 13 and 14, and the duration of symptoms was less than 12 hours in 78 percent of students. This instance of mass psychogenic illness was handled well as doctors, nurses and hospital staff recognized the likelihood of a psychogenic event early and provided calm reassurance to the sick students and their anxious relatives. They conducted appropriate but not excessive examinations and laboratory testing and immediately counteracted reports of a mysterious illness by the media and rumors of deaths in the community. Even though a later survey of the sick girls' guardians showed that 83 percent believed that the outbreak was due to some type of poisoning from the cake, by demonstrating the benign nature of the illness and the lack of any test abnormalities, most were adequately reassured. The responsible health officials appear to have followed the essential elements recommended to alleviate the wide-spread anxiety typically associated with an episode of mass psychogenic illness: (1) prompt recognition, (2) coordinated investigation, (3) effective stress and coping strategies, and (4) environmental modifications.

Laughing Mania

The capacity for psychogenic outbreaks to manifest in new and novel ways that are shaped by the social and cultural *zeitgeist* is no more evident than in the episodes of *endwara ya kucheka* or "the laughing trouble" [73]. Most of those affected were young girls. Since the mid-1960s, there have been many reports of people in parts of Central and Eastern Africa, exhibiting uncontrollable laughing in conjunction with bouts of weeping, screaming, twitching, shaking, trance-like states and histrionics. In August 1963, the *New York Times* reported on the epidemic:

> NAIROBI, Kenya, 8 Aug. Mass hysteria was suggested as the most likely answer today to the epidemic of laughing sickness along the shores of Lake Victoria.
> "I am certain that the outbreak does not have an organic basis," said Dr. Alexander Rankin, one of the medical investigators who uncovered the epidemic.
> "It must be purely mental," he said. "People in this area are highly superstitious."
> More than 1,000 Africans, most of them youngsters, have suffered fits of laughing and crying in the outbreak in the last 18 months.
> No deaths were reported, but the sickness has lasted from several hours to 16 days. The average has been 7 days. ...
> No teachers, policemen, village headmen or other relatively sophisticated adults in the area have contracted the symptoms.
> The epidemic has centered around the village of Bukoba in Tanganyika, on the western shores of Lake Victoria [74].

Since these reports first began to appear, there has been a deluge of similar cases [75–80]. While these outbreaks may seem bizarre, a closer look reveals an interesting pattern. Most are centered around missionary schools [75, 76, 78, 81]. These are classic symptoms of motor hysteria that are usually found in situations of longstanding repression, and this is exactly what investigators uncovered. Pediatrician G.J. Ebrahim of the Muhimbili Hospital in Tanganyika (now Tanzania) investigated several African incidents of Laughing Mania and attributed them to social and cultural tension. He wrote that African elders in the affected area were considered "all-powerful." Conflict arose when children began attending missionary schools which exposed them to radically different ideas that were often in conflict with traditional beliefs [81]. As to why outbreaks have taken the form of laughing, Central and Eastern Africa were the scenes of several major Christian revival movements during the first half of the twentieth century – movements that often included forms of worship that featured collective laughing [82]. By the early 1960s, missionary schools in the region were notorious for ignoring the cultural traditions of their students, while indoctrinating them in Western religious and cultural practices. This resulted in tension [83]. So why would elders allow their children to attend these schools if they were causing so much conflict? The answer is simple: they offered the only quality education in the area, and the parents wanted the best for their children. Missionary Jack Partain lived in Tanzania and described the conflict between Christianity and local beliefs, including divining the future and the power that ancestors hold over the living [84].

The Resurgence of Motor Hysteria in the West

In the twenty-first century, there has been a curious spike in the number of Western cases involving motor symptoms, especially in American schoolchildren. To put this trend in perspective, during the entire twentieth century, just four outbreaks of motor hysteria were recorded in United States schools. Since 2002, there have already been at least six. In 2002, 10 girls at a high school in North Carolina were stricken with mysterious seizures coinciding with the new school year. They also experienced fainting spells, dizziness, headaches, breathing problems, muscle twitching, tingling, and numbness. The school nurse was initially mystified, noting that while she had treated epileptic seizures before, the 'fits' were unlike anything she had ever seen [85]. As is common in the mass hysteria literature, the first person affected was a student of high status – a cheerleader. While most cases are confined to a single classroom, this was not the case as victims were spread throughout the ninth, tenth and eleventh grades. Neurological exams revealed that the seizures were psychogenic; they subsided within 4 months [85]. Five years later in 2007, the same pattern appeared. Nine girls and a female teacher at William Byrd High School in Virginia experienced twitching, headaches and dizziness. As with the North Carolina outbreak, investigators noted that those stricken were not confined to a single classroom but were spread throughout the school. The symptoms died down after several months and may have been driven by anxiety surrounding several local health crises including the death of an area student from a drug-resistant strain of Golden Staph [86].

In 2011, a strange malady affecting at least 14 girls and one boy swept through Leroy Central School in Western New York, generating international media attention. Symptoms included twitching muscles, facial tics, and garbled speech. The New York State Health Department eventually diagnosed the case as psychogenic. Once again, the affected students were spread throughout the school. While some parents disputed the mass hysteria diagnosis, one of the neurologists involved in treating 12 of the students, Laszlo Mechtler, observed that the girls were not exactly strangers: "Some of them were friends, some played on the same soccer team and all are in the same high school," he said [87]. He would also affirm that social media appeared to play a role in the outbreak. "It's remarkable to see how one individual post's something, and then the next person who posts something not only are the movements bizarre and not consistent with known movement disorders, but it's the same kind of movements. This mimicry goes on with Facebook" [86]. The news media also seems to have played a key role. "As soon as the media coverage stopped, they all began to rapidly improve and are doing very well," he wrote later (Mechtler L, McVige J, 2012 June 11, Dent Neurological Institute, Amherst, NY, and a "personal communication with Robert Bartholomew"). In 2012, a similar outbreak of vocal tics broke out at sister high schools in Massachusetts located just a few miles from one another. Nearly two dozen students were affected – all but one was female. The case was referred to in the media as contagious hiccups. The State's Health Department concluded that the case was an outbreak of mass hysteria, but kept their diagnosis hidden from the public until one of the authors (Bartholomew) filed for Freedom of Information documents [88]. Dewey High School in Oklahoma was the site of an outbreak of mysterious seizures among several female students in 2017. Symptoms included difficulty walking and talking. The State Health Department conducted a series of tests, eliminating the possibility of environmental contaminants and identifying conversion disorder as the cause [89–93].

While the form of mass psychogenic illness continues to change to reflect new anxieties, advice on dealing with outbreaks has remained unchanged since episodes in medieval nunneries: reassure those affected, separate them from the rest of the group, and send them home until the symptoms subside. Given the influence and proliferation of the Internet and social media networks, this latter advice may be unrealistic. Over the centuries, priests have been summoned to exorcize demons in a variety of challenging settings amid the widespread belief in witchcraft and sorcery. However, they were fortunate in one regard: they did not have to contend with Twitter, Facebook or mobile phones. In surveying the rich history of mass hysteria through the ages and its many forms, it would be wise not to underestimate the power of an idea, for the lesson from history is clear: we are all potential victims. Given the diverse manifestations of this phenomenon over the years, is it plausible to think that a group of diplomats in Cuba could have mistaken insect mating calls for a sonic attack and developed symptoms that reflected those fears? If history teaches us anything, it is that the human propensity for self-deception is only bound by imagination and plausibility. During the early stages of the outbreak, Cuban harassment using new technology was not only deemed to have been plausible, it was seen as the most likely explanation, triggering a series of remarkable events that became a self-fulfilling prophesy.

References

1. Geertz C. The interpretation of cultures. New York: Basic Books; 1973. p. 5.
2. Carson R. Silent spring. Boston: Houghton Mifflin; 1962.
3. Wessely S, Hyams K, Bartholomew RE. Psychological implications of chemical and biological weapons. BMJ. 2001;323(7318):878–9.

4. Lellman L. Suspicious incident forces subway's closing. Rutland Daily Herald (VT). 10 Oct 2001;Sect. A:3.
5. Meyer J. Subway spill sends jitters across world. Journal-Gazette. Fort Wayne (IN). 10 Oct 2001;Sect. 2:A.
6. Smothers M. Mysterious malady strikes kids on bus. Journal Star (Peoria, IL). 19 May 2000.
7. Bartholomew RE, Sirois F. Occupational mass psychogenic illness: a transcultural perspective. Transcult Psychiatry. 2000;37(4):495–524.
8. Bartholomew RE, Sirois F. Epidemic hysteria in schools: an international and historical overview. Educ Stud. 1996;22(3):285–311.
9. Abdul Rahman T. As I see it... will the hysteria return? The New Straits Times. 6 July 1987.
10. Hysterical pupils take schoolmates hostage. The New Straits Times. 19 May 1987. p. 1.
11. Hysteria: schoolgirls 'confess.' The New Straits Times. 21 May 1987. p. 3.
12. Hysteria blamed on 'evil spirits:' school head wants the ghosts to go. The New Straits Times. 23 May 1987. p. 7.
13. Council to meet over hysteria stricken girls. The New Straits Times. 24 May 1987. p. 4.
14. Seven girls scream for blood: hysterical outbursts continue. The New Straits Times. 25 May 1987. p. 4.
15. Interview: Fatimah, 'I only fulfilled my parents wishes.' The New Straits Times. 31 May 1987. p. 7.
16. 'I can't believe it, says pupil.' The New Straits Times. 31 May 1987. p. 7.
17. Bartholomew RE, Rickard B. Mass hysteria in schools: a worldwide history since 1566. Jefferson: McFarland; 2014. p. 87–8.
18. The feeling of suffocation and/or experiencing pressure on the chest are a common theme in 'night hag' tales of sleep paralysis in North America. Refer to: Hufford D. The terror that comes in the night. Philadelphia (PA): University of Pennsylvania Press; 1982.
19. Maines RP. The technology of orgasm: 'hysteria,' the vibrator, and women's sexual satisfaction. Baltimore: The John Hopkins University Press; 2001. p. 23.
20. Gordon BL. Medieval and renaissance medicine. New York: Philosophical Library; 1959. p. 562.
21. Perhaps the best known of these works is: Huxley A. The devils of Loudun. New York: Harper and Brothers; 1952.
22. Darnton R. The great cat massacre and other episodes in French cultural history. New York: Basic Books; 1984. p. 83–4.
23. Madden RR. Phantasmata or illusions and fanaticisms of protean forms productive of great evils, vol. 2. London: T.C. Newby; 1857.
24. Sluhovsky M. Believe not every spirit: possession, mysticism, & discernment in early modern catholicism. Chicago: University of Chicago Press; 2008. p. 238.
25. Robbins RH. The encyclopedia of witchcraft and demonology. New York: Crown; 1966.
26. Hecker JF. Epidemics of the middle ages. London: The Sydenham Society; 1844.
27. Guiley RE. The encyclopedia of witches and witchcraft. 2nd ed. New York: Checkmark Books; 1999. p. 7.
28. Görres J. La mystique divine, naturelle et diabolique, vol. 5. Paris: Poussielgue-Rusand; 1855. p. 328.
29. Calmeil LF. De la folie, consideree sous le point de vue pathologique, philosophique, historique et judiciaire, vol. 2. Paris: Baillere; 1945. p. 73.
30. Bekker B. Le monde enchanté, vol. 4. Amsterdam: Pierre Rotterdam; 1694. p. 517.
31. Wier J. Histoires, disputes et discours des illusions et impostures des diables, des magiciens infames, sorcières et empoisonneurs, vol. 1. Paris: Bureaux du Progrès Médical; 1886.
32. Montgeron L. La verité des miracles operés par l'intercession de M. de Paris, demontrée contre M. l'Archevêque de Sens. Utrecht: Chez les Libraires de la Compagnie;1737.
33. Bekhterev VM. Suggestion and its role in social life. 3rd ed. New Brunswick: Transaction Publishers; 1998.
34. Spiller G. Moral education in the boys' schools of Germany. In: Sadler ME, editor. Moral instruction and training in schools: report of an international inquiry, vol. 2. London: Longmans, Green & Company; 1908. p. 213–30.

35. Montgomery J. The education of girls in Germany: its methods of moral instruction and training. In: Sadler M, editor. Moral instruction and training in schools: report of an international inquiry, vol. 2. London: Longmans, Green & Company; 1908. p. 231–41.
36. Lukas J. Der schulmeister von sadowa. Kirchheim: Maniz; 1878.
37. Welch S. Subjects or citizens? elementary school policy and practice in Bavaria 1800–1918. Melbourne: University of Melbourne, Department of History Monograph 26;1998.
38. Burnham W. Suggestion in school hygiene. Pedagog Seminary. 1912;19:228–49.
39. Palmer D. Psychische seuche in der sbersten slasse einer sadchenschule. Centralbl f Nervenh u Psychiat. 1892;3:301–8.
40. Hirt L. Eine epidemie von hysterischen krampfen in einer Schleisischen dorfschule. Ztschr f Schulgsndhtspflg. 1893;6:225–9.
41. Rembold S. Acute psychiche contagion in einer madchenschule. Berl Klin Wochenschr. 1893;30:662–3.
42. Schutte P. Eine neue form hysterischer zustande bei schulkindern. Münch Med Woch. 1906;53:1763–4.
43. McEvedy CP, Griffith A, Hall T. Two school epidemics. BMJ. 1966;2:1300–2.
44. Moss PD, McEvedy CP. An epidemic of overbreathing among schoolgirls. BMJ. 1966;2:1295–300.
45. Goldberg EL. Crowd hysteria in a junior high school. J Sch Health. 1973;43:362–6.
46. Knight J, Friedman T, Sulianti J. Epidemic hysteria: a field study. Am J Public Health. 1965;55:858–65.
47. Olson WC. Account of a fainting epidemic in a high school. Psychol Clin (Phila). 1928;18:34–8.
48. Olczak P, Donnerstein E, Hershberger T, Kahn I. Group hysteria and the MMPI. Psychol Rep. 1971;28:413–4.
49. Teoh J, Yeoh K. Cultural conflict in transition: epidemic hysteria and social sanction. Aust N Z J Psychiatry. 1973;7:283–95.
50. Tam YK, Tsoi MM, Kwong B, Wong SW. Psychological epidemic in Hong Kong, Part 2, psychological and physiological characteristics of children who were affected. Acta Psychiatr Scand. 1982;65:437–49.
51. Wong SW, Kwong B, Tam YK, Tsoi MM. Psychological epidemic in Hong Kong, Part 1. Acta Psychiatr Scand. 1982;65:421–36.
52. Small GW, Propper M, Randolph E, Eth S. Mass hysteria among student performers: social relationship as a symptom predictor. Am J Psychiatry. 1991;148(9):1200–5.
53. Goh K. Epidemiological enquiries into a school outbreak of an unusual illness. Int J Epidemiol. 1987;16(2):265–70.
54. Michaux L, Lemperiere T, Juredieu C. Considerations psychpathologiques sur une epidemie d'hysterie convulsive dans un internat professionnel. Arch Fr Pediatr. 1952;9:987–90.
55. Schuler E, Parenton V. A recent epidemic of hysteria in a Louisiana high school. J Soc Psychol. 1943;17:221–35.
56. Taylor DC. Hysteria, belief, and magic. Br J Psychiatry. 1989;155:391–8.
57. St. Clare W. Gentleman's Magazine. 1787;57:268.
58. Lortie B. The envelope, please. Bull At Sci. 2002;58(6):9–10.
59. Taylor G. Irradiated-mail health woes 'mass hysteria' officials say. The Washington Times. 30 Jan 2002. p. 1.
60. Taylor G. Rumors spread hysteria epidemic. The Washington Times. 2002;2002:8.
61. Nemery B, Fischler B, Boogaerts M, Lison D, Willems J. The coca-cola incident in Belgium, June 1999. Food Chem Toxicol. 2002;40:1657–67.
62. Bartholomew RE, Evans H. Panic attacks: media manipulation and mass delusion. London: Sutton Publishing; 2004. p. 94.
63. The attack rate of the children, ages 10–17, was 16 percent in girls (28/179) and of 9 percent in boys (9/101) a ratio of 1.8 to 1.0.
64. Fifty-two percent of those affected were female, 37 percent were male, and in the remaining 11 percent the gender was not recorded.

65. Anonymous, Coke adds life, but cannot always explain it (Editorial). The Lancet. 1999;354(9174):173 (July 17).
66. Nemery B, Fischler B, Boogaerts M, Lison D. Dioxins, coca-cola, and mass sociogenic illness in Belgium. Lancet. 1999;354:77.
67. Mystery substance: 50 students treated for symptoms at Carterton. New Zealand Herald. 21 Sept 2018.
68. Johnston M. Ten sick children assessed in Wairarapa hospital after 'rotten eggs' smell hits Carterton school. New Zealand Herald. 21 Sept 2018.
69. Police say sulphur smell at Carterton school caused by compost from neighbouring property. Radio New Zealand (Wellington). 24 Sept 2018.
70. 19 pupils and teacher, hit by weird malady, fall out. The Bee (Danville, GA). 24 Apr 1936. p. 1.
71. Jones TF, Craig AS, Hoy D, Gunter EW, Ashley DL, Barr DB, et al. Mass psychogenic illness attributed to toxic exposure at a high school. N Engl J Med. 2000;342(2):96–100.
72. Tarafder BK, Khan MA, Islam MP, Mahmud SA, Sarker MH, Faruq I. Mass psychogenic illness: demography and symptom profile of an episode. Psychiatry J. 2016:1–5. https://doi.org/10.1155/2016/2810143.
73. Conley R. Laughing malady a puzzle in Africa. 1000 along Lake Victoria afflicted in 18 months – most are youngsters. The New York Times. 8 Aug 1963. p. 29.
74. Anonymous. The New York Times, 9 Aug 1963. p. 4.
75. Rankin AM, Philip PJ. An epidemic of laughing in the Buboka District of Tanganyika. Cent Afr J Med. 1963;9:167–70.
76. Kagwa BH. The problem of mass hysteria in East Africa. East Afr Med J. 1964;41:560–6.
77. Two schools close in Tanzania till siege of hysteria ends. The New York Times. 25 May 1966. p. 36.
78. Muhangi JR. Mass hysteria in an Ankole school. East Afr Med J. 1973;50:304–9.
79. Nkala G. Mass hysteria forces school closure. Middle East Intelligence Wire. 13 Mar 2000.
80. Owino W. Mass hysteria causes school's temporary closure. Pan African News Agency. 8 Mar 2000.
81. Ebrahim GJ. Mass hysteria in school children, notes on three outbreaks in East Africa. Clin Pediatr (Phila). 1968;7(7):437–8.
82. Pratney W. Revival. Lafayette: Huntington House; 1984. p. 267.
83. Murray TR, editor. International comparative education: practices, issues, & prospects. New York: Pergamon Press; 1991. p. 204.
84. Partain J. Christians and their ancestors: a dilemma in theology. Christian Century. 1986;103(36):1066–9.
85. Roach ES, Langley RL. Episodic neurological dysfunction due to mass hysteria. Arch Neurol. 2004;61(8):1269–72. See p. 1270
86. Harrison D. Expert: mystery illness is stress. The Roanoke Times. 18 Nov 2007.
87. 12 girls at NY high school develop involuntary tics; doc says it's 'mass psychogenic illness.' The Washington Post. 20 Jan 2012.
88. Bartholomew RE. Public health, politics and the stigma of mass hysteria: lessons from an outbreak of unusual illness. JRSM. 2016;109(5):175–9.
89. Letter from Kristy K. Bradley, State Epidemiologist, Oklahoma State Department of Health, to Robert Bartholomew. 6 Feb 2018.
90. Slanchik A. Dewey students suffering from similar symptoms, concerning parents. TV 6 News Report (Tulsa, OK). 3 Nov 2017.
91. Guillroy T. Female students allegedly paralyzed after seizures; parents concerned. TV 2 News Report (Tulsa, OK). 4 Nov 2017.
92. Vincent V. Letter from Dewey high school superintendent circa November 6, 2017, posted on the school's website.
93. Droege E. Dewey school illness: official reassures community. Bartlesville: Bartlesville Examiner-Enterprise; 2017.

Musical Illness and Telephone Sickness: An Early History of Sound and Suggestion

It's social effects were such as no other instrument whatever has produced. Its tones could… make women faint; send a dog into convulsions; make a sleeping girl wake screaming through a chord of the diminished seventh, and even cause the death of one very young [1].

–Karl Leopold Röllig on the glass armonica

There is no credible evidence to support the assertion that a sonic attack, either accidental or by design, ever took place against US or Canadian Embassy personnel in Cuba or American diplomats in China and Uzbekistan. The supposed result of these so-called attacks – brain injury from sound waves, is not only unlikely, it is impossible. Our ears are the 'canary in the coal mine' when it comes to the potential for sound waves to damage the brain. The cochlea of the inner ear would be damaged long before the brain is affected. To suggest that an acoustical device could be made that would selectively damage the brain without affecting hearing, ignores fundamental principles of biology and physics. Our ears have evolved to be highly sensitive to sound waves, while the brain is highly resistant to those same waves as it is shielded by dense bone. Despite initial claims to the contrary, there is no compelling evidence for white matter tract damage, concussion-like brain damage or hearing loss. There is only one plausible explanation capable of explaining the events in Cuba – an unfortunate series of events driven by mass suggestion, namely psychogenic illness and the redefinition of ever-present symptoms and sounds as sonic attack-related. There are many historical examples where sound waves have been erroneously attributed to health complaints, beginning with a device created by one of the founding fathers of the American Revolution, Benjamin Franklin.

The Curious Case of the Glass Armonica

In earlier times music was used to treat a range of conditions including what conventional medicine now considers to be psychosomatic illnesses. Hippocrates and his fellow Greek physicians recommended soothing music and bed rest to treat back

© Springer Nature Switzerland AG 2020
R. W. Baloh, R. E. Bartholomew, *Havana Syndrome*,
https://doi.org/10.1007/978-3-030-40746-9_6

pain and headache. During the Middle Ages, musicians in what is now Southern Italy played tunes to treat supposed victims of bites by tarantula spiders and an array of insects. As we will see in Chap. 9, episodes of Tarantism probably illustrate the classic nocebo-placebo effect with the expectation of illness after the real or imagined bite driving the symptoms, and the expectation of a cure after dancing to music, driving the recovery. The positive association between music and health almost completely reversed by the turn of the nineteenth century and many in the United States and Europe viewed exposure to music in a negative light. During this period, the "nerve paradigm of disease" dominated medical thinking whereby physical and mental illnesses were thought to stem from excess stimulation of nerves, including the auditory nerves from listening to too much music. By 1877, popular Canadian science writer Grant Allen asserted in his book *Physiological Aesthetics* that music was a major factor in the appearance of disease. He wrote that "auditory nerves are not liable to be scratched, burned, bruised, or attacked by chemical agents, but only to be wearied by overuse or jarred by discordant sounds" [2].

The initial link between music and illness began during the late eighteenth century. In 1787, Scottish physician James Adair wrote that some people have auditory nerves that are extremely sensitive to sound and can result in an assortment of symptoms [3]. In 1807, Austrian composer and physician Peter Lichtenthal concluded that musical stimulation could have potentially damaging consequences by stimulating the heart and blood vessels [4]. Females were believed to be especially susceptible to the harmful effects of music just as they were thought to be more sensitive to developing hysteria. In 1837, Irish physician James Johnson, doctor to William IV, claimed that music was harmful to the female constitution and could damage their delicate nervous systems. "The mania for music injurs the health and even curtails the life of thousands and tens of thousands annually, of the fair sex…. The consequence is, that the corporeal functions languish and become impaired…" [4, p 42]. Prague physician Leopold Raudnitz concurred with his assessment, writing in 1840 that "one finds a greater sensitivity for music among women than among men; since men's nerves have a far lower degree of sensitivity than those of women, whose nerves are very mobile and sensitive. Men are not as easily stimulated or excited as women. This is especially true in younger years when they are approaching maturity, when a lively sound, a quick and unexpected transition from one key to another can set women's nerve strength in remarkable motion" [5]. This widespread nineteenth century view is reflected in the popular 1825 book of advice to young women, *Domestic Duties, Or, Instructions to Young Married Ladies*. In it, Mrs. William Parkes warned that music could trigger miscarriages and cause infertility. She wrote about a woman who was so negatively affected by playing the harp that she "suffered fifteen successive miscarriages" [6]. Influential American physician George Beard, who popularized the term neurasthenia or "nervous exhaustion," believed that music could induce this condition on the nervous system [7]. Historian James Kennaway observes that the psychological influence of music may be a result of social delusions [4]. "It should also be remembered that it is quite possible that many of the accounts of music causing disease refer to real physical symptoms and suffering, albeit generally with a psychosomatic rather than direct physiological explanation" [8, p 128].

An instrument at the center of the controversy over music and health was the glass armonica invented by the famous American statesman Ben Franklin and unveiled in 1761. This same instrument was also referred to as the glass harmonica, although it had no connection with the mouth organ or harmonica. Franklin's device worked by spinning glass discs on a shaft driven by a flywheel. It quickly gained popularity and an estimated 5000 had been produced by the time of his death in 1790 [9]. For the first 30 years of its existence, the glass armonica enjoyed widespread popularity across North America and Europe. The German *Musical Almanac* wrote in 1787: "Of all musical inventions, the one of Mr. Franklin's has created the greatest excitement. Concerning the way of producing tones, it is an entirely new kind of instrument" [10, p 185]. The armonica was the musical darling of the late eighteenth century. However, near the end of the century it went from having been a therapeutic device to harming health. In other words, it went from being a placebo to a nocebo over a few decades. Franklin's invention was inspired by watching performances of musical glasses filled with varying amounts of water, which gave off different tones [1]. The glasses were played by tapping the containers with a stick or more commonly by rubbing the rim with a moistened finger. Music generated by rubbing one's fingers on the surface of drinking glasses already had a tradition of eliciting positive health effects. In *Deliciae Physicomathematicae* published in 1677, G.P. Hasdorfer writes about "an account of an experiment with four glasses, filled with brandy, wine, water and salt water or oil. The diverse sounds produced by the contrasting content of the glasses were thought not only to correspond to the emotions aroused by the four 'humours' of the human body, but even to have the power of alleviating or curing such disorders as a thickness of the blood" [11, p 488]. Throughout the eighteenth century, there were many musical performers who toured the continent using musical glasses, which were widely held to have "physiological and psychological influences on the listener" [1, 12, p 329].

Franklin's invention of the armonica was inspired by a performance using musical glasses and was initially reputed to have similar effects. In her memoir, Polish Princess Izabella Czartoryska wrote of an encounter with Franklin in 1772, who she claimed had miraculously healed her by playing the armonica. "I was ill, in a state of melancholia, and writing my testament and farewell letters. Wishing to distract me, my husband explained to me who Franklin was and to what he owed his fame... Franklin had a noble face with an expression of engaging kindness. Surprised by my immobility, he took my hands and gazed at me saying: *pauvre jeune femme*. He then opened a harmonium, sat down and played long. The music made a strong impression on me and tears began flowing from my eyes. Then Franklin sat by my side and looking with compassion said, 'Madam, you are cured.' Indeed that moment was a reaction to my melancholia. Franklin offered to teach me how to play the harmonium – I accepted without hesitation, hence he gave me twelve lessons" [13, p 362].

German physician Franz Mesmer used the armonica in his attempts to 'cure' people from various ailments with some success, highlighting the psychosomatic power of belief in the device. Mesmer discovered a power that he considered unique to humans called "animal magnetism." He believed that certain people, himself included, had a special power to influence the brain and cure a variety of diseases.

He could unleash the mysterious power simply by touching or gazing at the patient or by moving his hands over the surface of the body without touching it. He found that he could treat large numbers of patients at the same time by filling a tub with iron filings, from which protruded rods that the patients could hold onto to receive the stored magnetic energy – a tub full of 'animal magnetism.' Mesmer used background music sometimes provided by a glass armonica, as 'the great healer,' dressed in a lavender silk robe, walking among his thankful patients, touching them with a long, magnetized rod. In one incident that took place between 1778 and 1779, a doctor Le Roux observed how Mesmer was treating an army surgeon affected by gout, and how the haunting power of the music of the glass armonica suddenly and profoundly affected him. "Mr Mesmer then seated him near the harmonica; he had hardly begun to play when my friend was affected emotionally, trembled, lost his breath, changed color and felt pulled to the floor" [14, p 37].

But by the early decades of the nineteenth century, the glass armonica had all but disappeared from the public music scene amid a flurry of rumors and controversy. The instrument became a focal point of critics who feared that its music was harming audience members and the musicians themselves. It was said to have been especially harmful to the female nervous system. This led to a reaction by "well-bred women who would publicly swoon during a time when overly nervous or sensitive emotional 'hysteria' symbolized virtue, truth, and beauty" [14, p 7]. Heather Hadlock writes that these episodes of public swooning in reaction to the armonica, were likely a combination of habit and imagination, where women were "manufacturing the expected responses to it" [15, p 528]. As one writer observed in 1819, "When it was claimed that the armonica exerted a magical influence on the nerves, the instrument could not fail to captivate every sensitive soul. For any young lady of breeding it would have been most ill-advised, as soon as the glasses were even touched, not to fall into a tolerably convincing swoon.... Even ladies of mature age fancied themselves transported" [15, p 528].

Of all the instruments in use at the time, the armonica gained the reputation of being the most dangerous. This belief became a self-fulfilling prophecy. Stories of the harm posed by the instrument were fueled by the declining health of several prominent armonica players including the deaths of Marianne Davies in 1792 and Marianne Kirchgässner in 1808 [12]. Davies, the first person to master the instrument, gave concerts throughout Europe, to rave reviews. Despite its widespread use without any obvious health problems, amid a growing chorus of concern over its safety, by the turn of the century, Franklin's instrument had lost its luster. Its high-pitched sounds were soon blamed for an array of medical conditions arising from the damaged nervous system including general unwellness, fainting, convulsions, and mental health issues. It was said to be able to drive people to madness and was even attributed to marital disputes [12]. In his 1822 work, *De L'hypochondrie et Du Suicide*, French psychiatrist Jean-Pierre Falret (1794–1870) linked the armonica to taking one's life [8]. Players began to complain of dizziness, cramps, muscle spasms, and nervousness. Some researchers have suggested that lead from the glass was leaching into the skin of the players. However, this theory has been thoroughly discredited. The same health complaints were recorded by audience members, mostly female, who had no direct contact with the instrument. Furthermore, most cases of lead poisoning occur from eating or breathing it; absorption through the skin is difficult. Contemporary armonica historian and performer William Zeitler observes that all known eighteenth century armonicas were made of soda-lime glass and contained no lead, as this type of glass was more common and much less expensive. Even Franklin's device was made of soda lime, as was presumably the one he gifted to Marianne Davies [16, 17]. While some armonicas were painted, even if the paint contained lead, the practice at the time was to always paint the glass on the inside as the rubbing of wet fingers against the bare glass is necessary to make the high-pitched sound. Zeitler has even looked at the life expectancy of several prominent armonica players who were performing near the turn of the nineteenth century, and found that Davies and Kirchgässner were the exceptions; most lived well beyond the life expectancy of the period [18].

Part of the allure and panic over the appearance of the armonica, was its unique and eerie sound, falling between 1000 and 4000 Hertz. Kate Hepworth observes that these are "frequencies that the brain struggles to comprehend in terms of identification and location of sound." This gave the instrument its eerie, spooky, otherworldly qualities. As a result, the device was used to enhance phantasmagoria shows and seances [14]. From the Greek, *phantasma* (phantom) and *agoereuein* (to speak in public), these presentations were a form of horror theatre that gained popularity in Europe during the late eighteenth and nineteenth centuries. Medical historian Stanley Finger writes that the armonica's otherworldly quality was ideal for frightening audiences and conveying a supernatural presence during presentations, which typically included the projection of ghosts and demons on walls and the use of smoke to stoke emotions and create a supernatural atmosphere [19, pp 116–7].

German armonica player and composer Karl Leopold Röllig helped to fan fears surrounding Franklin's invention when in 1787 he cautioned people to avoid the device if they suffered from nervous complaints. He recommended that even healthy people should limit their time playing the instrument, and not to play late at night when its effects are enhanced. If this was not enough, he no doubt frightened many by asserting that armonica-induced illnesses were sometimes fatal. He offered himself as an example of what can happen when the device is played to excess. Röllig reported experiencing an array of symptoms that he attributed to the armonica, ranging from nervousness and muscle spasms to dizziness, tremors and terrifying hallucinations that involved seeing ghosts and hearing threatening noises. He claimed that these symptoms ceased when he stopped playing [19]. Röllig once famously wrote of the armonica's impact: "Its social effects were such as no other instrument whatever has produced. Its tones could…make women faint; send a dog into convulsions; make a sleeping girl wake screaming through a chord of the diminished seventh, and even cause the death of one very young [1].

German playwright Friedrich Rochlitz (1769–1842) helped to promote the scare when he observed that there was a shortage of armonica players, reinforcing a growing belief that the instrument's tone was leading to an array of nervous disorders and depression. He also believed that stringed instruments such as the harp and guitar produced a similar effect [19]. In 1798, he wrote that the main reason for the scarcity of armonica players was "the almost universally shared opinion that playing it is damaging to the health, that it excessively stimulates the nerves, plunges the player into a nagging depression and hence into a dark and melancholy mood… Many (physicians with whom I have discussed this matter) say the sharp penetrating tone runs like a spark through the entire nervous system, forcibly shaking it up and causing nervous disorders" [1, p 246]. A decade earlier, Johann Christian Muller (1776–1836) wrote an armonica instruction manual, warning of its potential dangers. "If you have been upset by harmful novels, false friends, or perhaps a deceiving girl then abstain from playing the armonica – it will only upset you even more. There are people of this kind – of both sexes – who must be advised not to study the instrument, in order that their state of mind should not be aggravated" [1, p 246]. Physician Anthony Willich observed that the armonica "induces a great degree of nervous weakness. And this effect is much accelerated by the acute and vibrating sounds of this instrument, by which the organs of hearing are intensely affected" [20, p 413].

Telephone Sickness

The development of new technologies has long been associated with an array of subjective illness complaints for which there is no corresponding cause-effect relationship. During the latter nineteenth century, the appearance of vague, fatigue-related conditions were attributed to the telegraph and steam power. During the early decades of the twentieth century, signals from commercial AM radio were blamed on everything from outbreaks of nausea to changing weather patterns [21, p 117]. Perhaps the most striking illustration of this trend was the reaction to Thomas Edison's invention of the incandescent light bulb in 1879. Historian Linda Simon writes that this new technology was so feared that 30 years later, just 10% of homes nationwide had electricity. Newspaper articles warned that reading in artificial light could cause blindness [22, pp 4–5]. In some instances, sound waves were viewed as the offending stimulus, as in the case of the telephone.

When on March 10, 1876, Alexander Graham Bell famously spoke into his talking device, "Mr. Watson, come here, I want to see you," his new invention of the telephone created great excitement. It also generated anxiety over its possible health effects. Even before Bell's device was successfully tested, people were concerned about the potential health risks of new, rapidly advancing technologies. These fears have often given rise to an array of subjective health complaints that parallel outbreaks of mass psychogenic illness. One example is the appearance of "telephone tinnitus" during the latter nineteenth century, which was attributed to long periods of listening on the phone. During September 1889, the author of an article in the *British Medical Journal* warned of this new malady that was said to be common among telephone operators. It was characterized by "nervous excitability, with buzzing noises in the ear, giddiness, and neuralgic pains." The condition was attributed to the sound waves. The author wrote about the cause as the "almost constant strain of the auditory apparatus…In some cases, also, the ear seemed to be irritated, by the constantly recurring sharp tinkle of the bell, or by the nearness of the sounds conveyed through the tube, into a state of oversensitiveness which made it intolerant of sound, as the eye when inflamed or irritable, becomes unable to bear the light" [23, p 672].

Another common condition of telephone operators was "sound shock:" widespread claims of serious ear damage resulting from excessive noise from the receiver. In 1926, ear specialist J.A. White of Richmond, Virginia, discussed the psychogenic nature of the condition of a young woman who answered the phone at a local department store. One day she received a call, picked up the receiver and upon hearing a noise, suffered vertigo and head pain. However, when Dr. White examined her, he could find no evidence of ear trauma [24]. In consulting other otologists, one wrote back that "he had seen patients, who claimed they had the ear damaged by violent vibration of the magnetized membrane of the telephone receiver, but he could find no real foundation for the complaint" [24, p 487]. One ear specialist told White that while some people claimed to have suffered concussions from exposure to loud telephone noises, "he had never seen a case where a concussion either from [a] telephone or other source had been responsible for a disturbance in the internal ear" as "this could only occur from a great trauma…[as] tremendous violence was necessary to produce concussion of the internal ear" [24, p 488]. Dr. White diagnosed the woman's condition as being "a hysterical manifestation" – what would be termed today as psychogenic. In 1926 – as today, a telephone cannot cause a concussion. The term "inner ear concussion" is poorly defined and is rarely used. It would refer to inner ear damage from major head trauma that actually damages the inner ear membrane. Sound at any level would not cause an inner ear concussion. Very loud sound greater than 140 decibels can damage the cochlear hair cells if the exposure is sustained, but there is no evidence that intense sound can damage the vestibular part of the inner ear, which is involved in the control of balance and eye movements. Early twentieth century claims that the condition of "acoustic shock" could be caused by a loud noise or listening to "crackling sounds" in the phone receiver – and was capable of producing a concussion, parallel contemporary claims that Cuban diplomats suffered concussion-like symptoms from being exposed to a sonic device.

A kindred condition considered to be of psychogenic origin was "traumatic" or "accident neurosis" which was common among German telephone operators. It is estimated that several thousand operators were affected. A typical case involved a woman operator in Göttingen, who was unable to work for nearly 2 months after receiving what she perceived to have been an electric shock in one of her ears. Within 6 months of returning to work, she experienced a second incident which was blamed on "crackling in the receiver as a result of atmospheric electricity" [25, p 201]. The malady broke out in epidemic proportions in Germany over the first two and a half decades of the twentieth century at a time when it was believed that answering calls for up to 8 hours a day would stress the vulnerable female nervous system. As one physician wrote in 1902, "What over-exertion of all mental faculties is required of a telephone operator!' 'Speaking, listening, connecting, in rapid unceasing succession the operator carries out her task, completely exhausted by the time she leaves the office…. Sleeplessness, or hearing telephone voices during her sleep – these are the first signs of severe nervousness" [25, p 204].

While stress, overwork, and fatigue were seen as major health concerns for phone operators, the focus of many physicians during this period was the reaction of the female nervous system to minor shocks and sounds heard over the phone. At the time, phones were equipped with buttons that the caller could press if they grew inpatient for service from an operator. Pressing the button drew the operator's attention by sending a mild current through the line. The result was an "unpleasant crackling noise or a slight shock" [25, p 205]. Beginning in the early 1920s, Ewald Stier was commissioned to study health problems of the German national phone system, leading him to call into question the very existence of 'telephone sickness' which he viewed as a form of "psychic infection." Of particular interest was the two-pronged attack on the malady as it lost its status as a medical condition: publicity surrounding the government's decision to no longer compensate for the 'disorder' and efforts by Stier to educate workers about the psychological origin of their complaints of electric shock [25]. These appear to have helped counter the nocebo effect in telephone operators. The appearance of health complaints in female German telephone operators that were attributed to electrical shocks and crackling sounds in the earpiece, coincided with the widespread belief that women were innately susceptible to psychosomatic illness as a result of anxiety, noise and overwork. An incident in 1902 illustrates this when a new telephone switchboard was installed at the headquarters of the Siemens Company in Berlin. In his history of the company, Georg Siemens recounts that initially the new operation went smoothly, but as the call volume got heavier, the female operators were unable to cope. "The calls piled up and the wrong connections multiplied, while the faulty cables added cross-talk to the confusion. By about 11 o'clock some 1000s of inherently nervous Berlin businessmen had become little short of raving mad, and the telephone operators had lost their heads. Suddenly one of the operators tore her 'phone set from her head and fell into hysterics, an example that was infectious. A few minutes later, the room was a mass of screaming and howling women, some of whom jumped up from their seats and rushed out. In the midst of the tumult the Director of Telegraphs stood with arms raised to the heavens wailing: 'My poor girls! My poor girls!'" [26, p 161].

Acoustic Shock Today

Even today, the diagnosis of 'acoustic shock' can be seen on medical certificates issued by Ear, Nose and Throat specialists, audiologists, general practitioners, and psychiatrists. The condition involves the appearance of an array of symptoms in phone users in response to exposure to brief, often loud, unexpected sounds – everything from fax tones to feedback noise and the human voice. However, there is overwhelming evidence that 'acoustic shock' is psychogenic. As Australian physician R.E. Hooper observes: "The relatively short duration of noise exposure, which in most cases involves sound levels that do not exceed statutory limits, together with variation in the onset of symptomatology, suggest that the condition is psychogenic" [27]. During the latter twentieth century as telephone use became routine, concern over 'acoustic shock' waned with one conspicuous exception: telephone operators in call centers or similar workplace environments. It was known for many years that people who routinely wore telephone headsets were subject to sudden random noises. Studies in the 1970s documented that workers in these environments were frequently exposed to noise transients lasting milliseconds to seconds in the 90- to 120-decibel range (acoustic incidents) but there was no identifiable change in hearing levels after such exposure [28]. Since 1991, most major manufacturers have incorporated an acoustic limiter in the electronics of their headsets so that any type of noise above 118 decibels is cut off and not transmitted to the ear. Some workers exposed to "acoustic incidents" complained of a range of symptoms including ear pain and fullness, ringing in the ears, dizziness and imbalance, anxiety and depression [29]. People reported sensations like being stabbed in the ear with an ice pick or like being electrocuted in the ear. In reaction, many operators threw off their headsets. The syndrome became known as "acoustic shock" and outbreaks were reported in countries around the world.

A major contemporary study of acoustic shock was carried out in Australia during the late 1990s. The most common immediate symptoms were ear pain (81%), tinnitus (50%) and imbalance (48%). In about 10%, the pain even involved the neck, jaw, and face, while a small number of affected people reported sensations of ear plugging and even blacking out. Other symptoms developed later, including anxiety, depression, sensitivity to previously tolerated sounds, hypervigilance, fear, and anger. Of 103 people reporting symptoms of acoustic shock in the Australian study, 91 were women (89%), whereas females represented 74% of the call center workforce. In a study from Denmark that looked at acoustic shock from fourteen different call centers, many had no cases of acoustic shock, while in one center, 22% of callers reported experiencing it [29]. There was a significant correlation between stress, smoking, neck and shoulder pain, and developing acoustic shock. Those with multiple episodes tended to have the most severe symptoms.

With the high rate of tinnitus and ear pain associated with acoustic shock, it was natural to consider damage to the middle or inner ear as a cause for the condition, but numerous studies failed to identify objective evidence of ear damage. Furthermore, it would be difficult to explain the many symptoms of acoustic shock based on ear damage alone. Studies exposing normal subjects to brief moderate intensity sounds similar to those observed with acoustic shock did not produce any signs of ear damage. Episodes of acoustic shock, like outbreaks of mass psychogenic illness, tend to occur in clusters. Conspicuously, the condition, while common in some centers and geographical areas, was absent in other centers and areas with identical telecommunications equipment. The most likely explanation is that the sudden, unexpected noise triggered anxiety, particularly in people with a propensity for anxiety and phobias. These subjects had a heightened sensitivity to sound and increased startle responses to noise, and just as with pain, fear-avoidance behavior can occur with loud sounds [30]. A vicious cycle develops whereby anxiety increases sensitivity to noise and loud noise increases anxiety. Interestingly, central auditory hypersensitivity occurs with several conditions associated with altered serotonin metabolism in the brain including migraine, post-traumatic stress disorder, anxiety, and depression. British neurologist Jon Stone observed that symptoms of acoustical shock in professional telephone operators occurred with similar frequency in 'Havana Syndrome,' including headache, dizziness, imbalance, persistent ear pain, sensitivity to noise, tinnitus, and anxiety [31].

Some people claim that modern mobile phones make them sick, but instead of blaming sound, they blame electromagnetic waves. When mobile phones first came into general use there were dire predictions that the electromagnetic waves associated with them would increase the risk of brain cancer just as smoking increases the risk of lung cancer. But over time brain cancer rates remained steady despite the universal use of mobile phones. Other people attributed tinnitus, dizziness, and headaches to the electromagnetic waves, but just as with brief sounds, there is no scientific evidence that electromagnetic fields associated with mobile phones can damage the ear or brain [32, 33]. Double-blind studies have shown that people who claim they experience symptoms from exposure to electromagnetic fields are unable to detect the presence of these fields and sham exposure to electromagnetic fields causes symptoms as frequently as real exposure [34, 35]. Studies that assess people's expectations prior to being exposed to sham or real electromagnetic fields show that the so-called nocebo effect plays a key role in determining whether symptoms develop or not. If people expect to have symptoms, they are much more likely to have them.

The media plays an important role in shaping expectations. Media warnings about the adverse effects of modern life may become self-fulfilling. In a study on the impact of exposure to sham electromagnetic fields conducted in London, 147 healthy people were randomly assigned to watch a television documentary about the health effects of electromagnetic fields or a control documentary on mobile phones that did not mention health or electromagnetic fields [36]. Participants were told, "This project will assess whether a new type of electromagnetic field, which will be used in future mobile phones and WiFi systems, can cause short-term physical symptoms such as fatigue or headaches" [36, p 207]. After watching the documentaries, subjects were fitted with a headband and an attached antenna and told that the device was meant to bring the signal as close to them as possible. They were then told that they would be exposed to the electromagnetic field for 15 minutes and that they should watch for any symptoms that might develop during that time. They could terminate exposure if the symptoms became too strong. Eighty-two of the 147 participants (54%) reported symptoms which they attributed to the imaginary electromagnetic field exposure. Subjects who watched the documentary warning about health effects were much more likely to have symptoms. Men and women were equally affected. Those who had watched and attributed their symptoms to the sham exposure were significantly more likely to think they had increased sensitivity to electromagnetic fields than those who had symptoms but watched the control documentary.

References

1. Finger S. Doctor Stanley's medicine. Philadelphia: University of Pennsylvania Press; 2006. p. 245.
2. Allen G. Physiological aesthetics. New York: D. Appleton & Company; 1877. p. 98.

3. Adair JMA. Philosophical and medical sketch of the natural history of the human body and mind. Bath: R. Cruttwell; 1787.
4. Kennaway. Bad vibrations: the history of the idea of music as a cause of disease. London: Taylor & Francis; 2016. p. 35.
5. Raudnitz L. Die musik als heilmittel. Prague: Gottlieb Haase Söhne; 1840. p. 40–1.
6. Parkes W. Domestic duties, or, instructions to young married ladies, on the management of their households. London: Longman, Hurst, Rees, Orme, Brown, and Green; 1825. p. 296.
7. Thompson H. Some 19th-century physicians thought music could infect the brain. Smithsonian Magazine. 22 Jun 2015 . https://www.smithsonianmag.com/smart-news/19th-century-physicians-thought-music-was-disease-180955662/. Accessed 15 Mar 2018.
8. Kennaway J. Historical perspectives on music as a cause of disease. In: Alternmuller E, Finger S, Boller F, editors. Progress in brain research 2016: music, neurology, and neuroscience: historical connections and perspectives. Amsterdam: Elsevier; 2015. p. 127–45.
9. Franklin's Glass Armonica, The Franklin Institute. Accessed 21 Nov 2018 at: https://www.fi.edu/history-resources/franklins-glass-armonica.
10. Meyer V, Allen KJ. Benjamin Franklin and the glass armonica. Endeavour. 1988;12(4):185–8. p185.
11. King AH. The musical glasses and the glass harmonica. In: Proceedings of the Royal Music Association. London: Whitehead & Miller; 1946. p. 97–122. See 99, citing a passage from G.P. Hasdorfer, 1677, *Deliciae physicomathematicae,* p488.
12. Gallo DA, Finger S. The power of a musical instrument: Franklin, the Mozarts, Mesmer, and the glass armonica. Hist Psychol. 2000;3(4):326–43.
13. Lipowski ZJ. Benjamin Franklin as a psychotherapist: a forerunner of brief psychotherapy. Perspect Biol Med. 1984;27:361–6.
14. Hepworth KM. Eighteenth century women and the business of making glass music. California Polytechnic State University, San Luis Obispo, CA, Bachelor of Arts, (Department of History), 2017.
15. Hadlock H. Sonorous bodies: women and the glass harmonica. J Am Musicol Soc. 2000;53(3):507–42.
16. Mead C. Angelic music: the story of Ben Franklin's glass Armonica. New York: Simon & Schuster; 2017. p. 110–76.
17. Zeitler W. The glass armonica: the music and the madness. San Bernardino: Musica Arcana; 2013.
18. Zeitler W. The glass armonica: Benjamin Franklin's magical musical invention. 2009. http://www.glassarmonica.com/armonica/lead_poisoning.php. Accessed 11 Nov 2018.
19. Finger S, Zeitler W. Benjamin Franklin and his glass armonica: from music as therapeutic to pathological. In: Alternmuller WE, Finger S, Boller F, editors. Progress in brain research 2016: music, neurology, and neuroscience: historical connections and perspectives. Amsterdam: Elsevier; 2015. p. 93–125.
20. Willich AF. Lectures on diet and regimen: being a systematic inquiry into the most rational means of preserving health and prolonging life. together with physiological and chemical explanations, calculated chiefly for the use of families; in order to banish the prevailing abuses and prejudices in medicine. London: T.N. Longman & Paternoster Row;1901.
21. Rubin GJ, Burns M, Wessely S. Possible psychological mechanisms for 'wind turbine' syndrome. On the windmills of your mind. Noise Health. 2014;16(69):116–22. https://doi.org/10.4103/1463-1741.132099.
22. Simon L. Dark light: electricity and anxiety from the telegraph to the x-ray. Orlando: Harcourt; 2004.
23. The telephone as a cause of ear troubles. BMJ. 1889;2:671–2.
24. White JA. The telephone and the ear. Laryngoscope. 1928;38(7):486–92. See p486.
25. Killen A. From shock to schreck: psychiatrists, telephone operators and traumatic neurosis in Germany, 1900-26. J Contemp Hist. 2003;38(2):201–20.
26. Siemens G. History of the house of Siemens. New York: Arno Press; 1977.
27. Hooper R. Acoustic shock controversies. J Laryngol Otol. 2014;128:S2–9.

28. Alexander RW, Koenig AH, Cohen H. The effects of noise on telephone operators. J Occup Med. 1979;21(1):21–5.
29. McFerran DJ, Baguley DM. Acoustic shock. J Laryngol Otol. 2007;121:301–5.
30. Jüris L, Andersson G, Larsen HC, Ekselius L. Psychiatric comorbidity and personality traits in patients with hyperacusis. Int J Audiol. 2013;52:230–5.
31. Stone J, Popkirov S, Carson AJ. Letter. JAMA. 2018;320(6):602–3. https://doi.org/10.1001/jama.2018.8706.
32. Oftedal G, Wilen J, Sandström M, Mild K. Symptoms experienced in connection with mobile phone use. Occup Med (London). 2000;50(4):237–45.
33. Roosli M, Moser M, Baldinini Y, Meier M, Braun-Fahrländer C. Symptoms of ill health ascribed to electromagnetic field exposure – a questionnaire survey. Int J Hyg Environ Health. 2004;207(2):141–50.
34. Rubin GJ, Munshi D, Wessely S. Electromagnetic hypersensitivity: a systematic review of provocation studies. Psychosom Med. 2005;67(2):224–32.
35. Rubin GJ, Everitt BS, Wessely S. Are some people sensitive to mobile phone signals? Within participants double-blind randomized provocation study. BMJ. 2006;332(7546):886–91.
36. Witthöft M, Rubin GJ. Are media warnings about the adverse health effects of modern life self-fulfilling? An experimental study on idiopathic environmental intolerance attributed to electromagnetic fields (IEI-EMF). J Psychosom Res. 2013;74(3):206–12.

Modern-Day Acoustical Scares: From 'The Hum' to 'Wind Turbine Syndrome'

7

Where we have strong emotions, we're liable to fool ourselves.

–Carl Sagan [1]

The Cuban 'sonic attack' saga has many antecedents. One prominent example involves claims surrounding a mysterious humming sound that has been reported at numerous locations around the world. Since the early 1980s, several illness clusters have been associated with this sound. Government-funded studies of what has been dubbed 'the Hum,' have been conducted in Taos, New Mexico, Kokomo, Indiana, Windsor, Canada, and London, England. In each instance, investigators have either failed to locate the source or identified mundane origins. Other outbreaks of illness have been reported in groups of people living near wind turbines. Those affected are convinced that the culprit is low-frequency noise from the blades which turn to generate electricity. Before we explore these fascinating case studies, we will begin this chapter with the strange case of the humming giraffes.

The Devon Zoo Giraffe Saga

Outbreaks of mass psychogenic illness have taken many forms because episodes are driven by beliefs that are deemed to be plausible at a particular time and place. A good illustration of the pivotal role that plausibility plays can be seen in recent claims that humming sounds generated by giraffes at a British zoo were causing nearby residents to fall ill. Beginning in the fall of 2013, residents living near the giraffe enclosure of the Paignton Zoo in Devonshire, England, began to complain that a mysterious hum was making them ill – specifically, an oil gas boiler situated near the giraffe enclosure. In August 2014, 20 residents signed a petition and handed it to zoo authorities asking them to address the issue. Working with experts from the Environmental Health Department, they investigated and eliminated the boiler as the cause of the mysterious sound, and the zoo in general [2]. Then in 2015, the

© Springer Nature Switzerland AG 2020
R. W. Baloh, R. E. Bartholomew, *Havana Syndrome*,
https://doi.org/10.1007/978-3-030-40746-9_7

number of complaints about the mysterious humming at the zoo exploded, coinciding with widespread speculation that giraffes communicate through low-frequency humming after European scientists published a study which concluded that giraffes communicate by humming [3]. Prior to 2013, there are no known reports of giraffe humming causing people to become ill, be it from zoo staff around the world or neighbors living nearby. But by 2016, 165 residents living in the vicinity of the Paignton zoo signed another petition complaining that the mysterious humming was coming from the giraffe enclosure and was causing them to become sick. Symptoms included headaches, irritation, tremors, insomnia, heart palpitations, and a general state of ill health. One resident described the noise as resembling "a distant engine or washing machine." Others said it was "a persistent low level hum." Gillian Watling claimed that at night the noise created "waves passing down the muscles in my back, buttocks, thighs and calves." She likened the sensation to "the feeling you get standing next to a large bass speaker that is playing music very loudly at a rock concert." In response, the Torbay Council sent officers to the site but they were unable to detect any unusual noises at the enclosure or nearby. The Council even investigated the possibility that the noise was coming from a nearby factory but they could find nothing out of the ordinary in relation to low-frequency noise [4]. Reports of the 'Zoo Hum' spiked in 2016 shortly after a flurry of international news reports that biologists had discovered that giraffes communicate by humming as the physical construction of their long necks make it difficult to produce conventional vocalizations [5]. One of the researchers who identified the giraffe hum, Angela Stöger of the University of Vienna in Austria, said the hum was barely audible at 92 Hertz, making it highly unlikely it was what local residents were reporting as nearby residents would not be able to hear it. "Even giraffe keepers and zoo managers stated that they have never heard these vocalizations before," she said. As to why they hum only at night, it is believed that it is a means of reassuring their comrades in the dark that they are nearby [6]. In the original giraffe hum study, scientists recorded the animals for over 900 hours and were only able to identify sixty-five separate incidents involving hums. A zoo spokesperson observed: "These were very short calls, lasting a matter of seconds at most, which is not consistent with the sounds reportedly heard by the neighbour" [7].

The Hummers

There is a history of mysterious humming sounds inducing sickness, especially in Western countries since the late 1970s, coinciding with the rise of heightened environmental concerns and legislation. These waxing, waning outbreaks have gained considerable media attention, to the point where they have become part of regional folklore. Expectation plays a powerful role in these illness clusters associated with ambiguous sounds. News reports about these events have fueled many ongoing Hum scares, but only in recent times has it been associated with illness and irritation. There have been accounts of unidentified humming, buzzing and droning sounds as early as the eighteenth century. In 1769, Gilbert White, in his natural history of

Selbourne, England, described it as: "Humming in the air. There is a natural occurrence to be met with upon the highest part of our downs in hot summer days which always amuses me without giving me any satisfaction as to the cause of it; and that is the loud humming as of bees in the air, though not one insect is to be seen. The sound is distinctly to be heard the whole common through. Any person would suppose that a large swarm of bees was in motion and playing above his head" [8, p 98].

Between 1878 and 1879, the *Manchester City News* published a series of articles on the local phenomena. Many reports during the era were concentrated in the United Kingdom and seemed to have a musical quality. Nineteenth century British reports of the mysterious sound were commonly referred to as the "Hummadruz," a combination of the words 'hum,' 'drone' and 'buzz.' On May 18, 1878, local resident R.E. Bibby wrote: "The phenomena itself I have heard and listened to hundreds of times, and in common with my neighbours, with whom it was a sort of village wonder, vainly attempted to get at a solution of the mystery." The sound was described as "a low drone, or humming noise, which on calm days, particularly in clear weather, could be heard over the entire districts east and south of Manchester; the neighbourhoods of Gorton, Rusholme, and Longsight being places where I have noted them most frequently. … .Commonly speaking, the sounds were continuous, but at times the crescendos and diminuendos partook much of the character of the Aeolian harp, and were quite as musical" [8, pp 47–48]. *Samuel Hewitt* wrote to the paper to report having heard the Hummadruz on several occasions. He stated that 1 day he set off to find the source, only to come upon "a large pit, the surface of the water in which was covered by a multitude of frogs, whose croaking produced the strange sounds that had previously puzzled me" [8, p 62]. Another resident, Arlunydd Glan Conway, wrote that he too had heard the sound near Llyn Geirionydd. "It was about four o'clock in the afternoon when my attention was attracted by a continuity of musical minor murmuring strains, resembling the minor notes produced by the rain-wind playing sadly through the window sashes, and sometimes like the musical tones of the telegraph wires played upon by a whistling north-easter or south-wester." After packing up his traps and heading home, "this 'humadruzz' or humabuzz never left me until I left the moorland top. Before doing so I stooped and examined the dry wiry grass of the mountain, and to my surprise I found an infinitude of life everywhere, in the shape of small winged insects, producing these wild, weird, minor Eolian-harp kind of strains" [8, pp 62–63]. A curious aspect of the Manchester area Hummadruz and other mysterious sounds of this period are the descriptions: eighteenth and nineteenth century accounts are overwhelmingly recorded as pleasant and are conspicuously devoid of annoyance and medical complaints. Up until about 1980, twentieth century reports are typically described as annoying and irritating, but aside from insomnia, health problems attributed to the sound are absent. For instance, "the Kent Hum" in England had been reported since the late 1940s and peaked in the early 1960s, yet early news reports are devoid of health issues [9, 10].

During the 1970s, complaints of irritation begin to appear *en masse* and were soon followed by health issues near the end of the decade. The first major reporting on the Hum in the contemporary media occurred in 1977 when the British *Sunday Mirror* published a series of reports on cases in the United Kingdom and received an astounding 768 letters from readers claiming to have heard a similar sound [11]. Illness clusters associated with mysterious humming, buzzing, droning sounds began to appear around 1980, when residents living in Largs, Scotland, began complaining of an eerie low level hum that was making them sick. Reports continue to the present-day [12]. Symptoms include an array of ambiguous conditions and sensations from the perception of a vague vibrating sensation, to nose pressure, chest tightness, ear pain, insomnia, and general unwellness. A description by one resident, Georgie Hyslop, underscores the range of complaints: "If it's not too bad, it's a bit of a headache. As it gets worse it progresses to an ache across the sternum, like a tight band across my chest. My ears pop, and I get stabbing pains, vertically in my head. I get nosebleeds. My short-term memory goes, I feel nauseous and sometimes I am violently sick" [13]. Popular folk explanations for the 'Largs Hum' have included radio, radar and telecommunications towers. Some believe that the sound originates from submarines communicating with low-frequency sound waves; others suspect that it is generated from a natural gas pipeline [14–21]. Around the same time that health concerns were being raised in Largs, similar health complaints were being raised about the 'Bristol Hum' in southwest England which included complaints of headaches [22].

By the early 1990s, residents of Taos, New Mexico began complaining of a humming sound in their homes, particularly in the evening around sundown [23]. Taos is a small mountain desert community about 2 hours north of Albuquerque. If they went outside, the sound would typically disappear. It was common for one spouse to hear the sound while the other spouse sitting nearby heard nothing. Some described it like a diesel engine idling in the distance while others compared it to a whir or buzzing rather than a hum, but all agreed that the sound was annoying and persistent. Even more disturbing, many of the hearers claimed that the sound made them sick including headaches, dizziness, sleep disturbance, fatigue, ear pressure and loss of libido. It affected about 2% of the population, mostly between ages 30 and 59; men and women were equally affected [24]. Residents of the community were so alarmed by the mysterious noise that in 1993, they pleaded with Congress to send researchers to investigate the source of the humming. Congress took the issue seriously and funded a study. A team of 12 researchers from Los Alamos National Laboratory at the University of New Mexico, the Sandia National Laboratories and regional experts visited Taos to solve the mystery, but after spending a few weeks in the community, they were stumped. Investigators could find no source for the sound or explain why people were becoming sick [25]. After continuously monitoring the community during which time residents claimed to be hearing the hum, the only unusual readings were elevated electromagnetic fields which were likely from local power lines [26]. The researchers said they could not rule out the possibility that some people were especially sensitive to electromagnetic noise from electric household devices, microwave ovens and mobile phones [27]. The negative findings led some to speculate that the government was the source of the noise, possibly covering up testing of a new secret weapon in the vicinity.

As publicity surrounding the Taos Hum went national, authorities began receiving calls from across the United States, and the world, from people claiming that they had also heard what they called 'the Hum.' An early well-documented occurrence of 'the Hum' was in Bristol, England in the late 1960s and early 1970s [28]. Dubbed 'The Bristol Hum,' about 800 people in this coastal city complained of hearing the noise which they attributed to insomnia, and more recently, sickness in some. As in Taos, about 1 in 50 people reported hearing the sound, descriptions of which varied from a low-pitched hum to a higher pitched whir or buzzing. Two suicides were even attributed to the strange sound. In the late 1960s, scientists at London University flippantly suggested that hum hearers should try wearing an aluminum helmet to block out the sound, which was blamed on a variety of sources including traffic noise, industrial machinery, oscillation in the ocean bed and even the mating calls of fish. More recently, people even suggested that the noise was coming from wind farms in the Bristol area, ignoring the fact that these farms did not exist in the 1960s and 1970s when the problem was first noticed. How do we explain that only a small percentage of people can hear the sound? While health professionals have dismissed it as ringing in the ears or tinnitus, why would it only be heard in certain locations? Adding to the confusion, sporadic spates of hearing 'the Hum' sound have been recorded in Bristol for 50 years. There are some periods with few reports followed by a flurry of complaints. The experiences of Bristol resident Jamie Brightmore are typical. Between 2013 and 2017, she heard it on an irregular basis, although it was present most of the time. She did not hear it on trips to New York and France, but it was discernable in parts of London [29].

Jamie's account provides a clear description of what hummers (a common term used for people who hear the hum) experience in dealing with the recurring sound. They want to figure it out. They are sure it is real since they hear it and are frustrated when people are skeptical and suggest that it is all in their heads. But there are inconsistencies in the reports; most argue that it is low frequency, others speculate that it is most likely high frequency, yet they use examples such as a motor running, diesel truck idling, whirring or buzzing, which are mid-frequency sounds. Some people like Jamie report that 'the Hum' can be masked by background sounds such as a fan or refrigerator, suggesting that it is at least mid-frequency and not very loud. Masking sounds are commonly used to manage tinnitus which is usually high frequency, but if it was tinnitus, why didn't Jamie hear the sound while traveling? Ultrasound and barely audible frequencies from the duct systems in certain buildings have been proposed as a mechanism for 'the Hum' but, with rare exception researchers have not found evidence for sound resonating within buildings. Recently, hummers from all around the world have recorded their sounds and posted them on the internet. After listening to several of these recordings, it is obvious that they are not very loud and a wide range of sounds are being heard. Most of them are not much different from sounds we hear on a daily basis. It is difficult to see a pattern and clearly, the sounds have different frequencies and loudness. Could it be that these people are simply hearing normal background noises and that they become preoccupied with them? Many people prefer to have a fan on at night since the constant sound of the fan makes background noise in the environment less bothersome and less likely to interrupt sleep. Interestingly, environmental sounds are more distressing in quiet, rural areas, presumably because of the marked contrast between absolute quiet and the sounds.

In his article "The Hum: An Anomalous Sound Heard Around the World," University of Oklahoma Geophysicist David Deming reported that he too was a hummer: "Hearers typically go through phases. At first, they search for the source of the noise inside their homes. Internal sources are usually eliminated by shutting off all electrical power to the home. The next phase is to conduct searches for the source of the sound by walking or driving through neighborhoods late at night or early in the morning. These searches are always in vain; the source of the Hum is never found" [11, p 576]. Deming noted that the hum was often accompanied by a sense of vibration with some people even reporting that the doors and windows shake. He wrote, "There have been times in Norman, Oklahoma, when I would have sworn that my entire bed was vibrating, yet no objective movement can be seen or felt" [11, p 577]. This sense of vibration must be entirely subjective since attempts to objectively record hum vibrations have been consistently negative. Deming suggested that 'the Hum' might not be an acoustic sound at all but rather a low-frequency vibration generated by electromagnetic radiation at radio frequencies. So-called radiofrequency radiation sickness syndrome, with symptoms similar to those suffered by hummers, was first described by the Soviets in the 1950s and is even more controversial than hum sickness. It is supposed to result from chronic, low-intensity exposure to electromagnetic radiation at radio frequencies. Deming and others have suggested that 'the Hum' might be caused by a network of Navy aircraft developed in the 1960s that use very low-frequency (VLF) radio waves to communicate with submarines [11, 30]. VLF radio waves require massive antennae and high energy that can cover the globe and penetrate just about any surface including hundreds of feet of water to reach submarines. Possibly a small percentage of the population can hear these VLF waves.

In some hum occurrences the sounds were traced to a likely source. In the mid-1980s, people living near the sea in Sausalito, California reported hearing a hum that seemed to be coming from the ocean on summer nights [31]. Descriptions varied from the drone of a B-29 bomber to a giant electric shaver. People living in houseboats in the marina were particularly bothered by the sound, complaining that it kept them up at night. They sought out marine biologists at the local aquarium who traced the source to the mating calls of singing toadfish. The sound was able to penetrate the steel hulls of the houseboats. In 2012, people in West Seattle, Washington, 800 miles north of Sausalito, complained of a loud hum coming from the sea also keeping them up at night. Recordings of the sound were made and it too was identified as that of the singing toadfish [31].

A study funded by the Canadian government of 'The Windsor Hum' in Ontario Province concluded that the source of the sound was mundane: nearby blast furnaces [32]. While contemporary media reports trace the origin of this hum to 2011, a search of historical newspapers reveals complaints of a mysterious noise in the vicinity of Windsor as far back as 1959, yet this report is devoid of health complaints, only annoyance [33]. Only in recent years has 'The Hum' become the focus of significant public concern [34]. People in Windsor have been complaining of hearing a sound like a fleet of diesel engines idling. Others report that it can rattle windows and scare pets. Symptoms include nausea, headaches, insomnia and anxiety [35–38]. Windsor resident, Sabrina Wiese says 'the Hum' has destroyed her quality of life. "You know how you hear of people who have gone out to secluded places to get away from certain sounds or noises and the like? I've wanted to do that many times in the past year or so because it has gotten so bad. Imagine having to flee all you know and love just to have a chance to hear nothing humming in your head for hours on end" [34]. Researchers from the University of Windsor and Western University in London, Ontario traced a possible source to the sound of blast furnaces run by United States Steel operating on Zug Island in the Detroit River. This has led to international intrigue with US Steel denying that their furnaces could be the cause of the origin, and Ontario officials claiming that they need more time and cooperation with the Americans to identify the source. Meanwhile 'the Hum' has also been heard in McGregor, Ontario, 20 miles to the south and from near Cleveland, 90 miles away. Professor Colin Novac, the chief investigator on the Windsor study noted, "It's like chasing a ghost". Tim Carpenter, a retired consulting engineer specializing in machine vibrations, has been studying the 'Windsor Hum' for years and observes that even if the original cause was found and eliminated, it could be replaced by other mechanical sounds entering the spectrum of hearable sounds [34].

Between 1999 and 2002, about 100 residents of the town of Kokomo in Central Indiana, became convinced that their illnesses were linked to a mysterious intermittent low-pitched rumbling or humming sound. Among the symptoms were headaches, dizziness, muscle and joint pain, fatigue, insomnia; even nosebleeds and diarrhea [39–47]. Local resident Maria McDaniel and her family attributed 'the Kokomo Hum' to everything from nausea to joint pain, irritability and disorientation. She said that family members often felt as if they were walking around with a hangover. Evelyn Floyd believes that the 'Kokomo Hum' was responsible for ongoing medical problems that include headaches, muscle cramps, memory loss, depression and a variety of aches and pains. In one incident, she described "a sudden vibration, shooting up my legs and spine, that shook me like a rag doll" [48]. A study failed to find a link between the sound and symptoms [49].

LaQuita Zimmerman, a lifelong resident of Kokomo said, "I think we all know something was starting to go drastically wrong about 2 years ago. It went from a headache to a never-ending headache" [50]. Maria McDaniels who lived several miles from Zimmerman, noted that she, her two sons and her husband experienced headaches, sleep problems and diarrhea after hearing the noise. "We just noticed a low hum – a drone in the background. It seemed to increase in intensity in the wee hours of the night." Others reported a range of symptoms caused by sound including dizziness, extreme fatigue, joint and muscle pain, and nose bleeds. Indiana senator Richard Lugar's office received more than 80 letters complaining about 'the Hum.' The *Kokomo Tribune* reported that most of the people who heard it had visited a doctor on multiple occasions for health problems related to the sound and more than a third underwent neurological testing. Doctors mostly attributed the symptoms to anxiety. A 2002 study financed by the city of Kokomo identified the most likely source of the humming: massive fans at the Daimler-Chrysler car manufacturing plant. Despite cooperation by plant officials in abating the sound, people continued to hear 'the Hum' [49].

In 2012, school teacher Glen MacPherson, living in Gibsons, British Columbia, a small town in western Canada, began hearing droning sounds of what he initially thought were seaplanes taking off and landing. After a week or so he realized that the sound could not be coming from planes since it went away when he went indoors. The noise usually occurred in the evening. To investigate the source, he systematically turned off appliances, then shut off the power to the house. Much to his surprise, the sound became louder. Oddly, he noticed that the humming could be briefly shut off if he turned his head sharply or exhaled, but then it quickly returned. MacPherson considers himself a hum hearer and not a hum sufferer since he has not developed symptoms other than annoyance. Having a background in computer science, he initially reported his personal experience on the internet and decided to develop a website for Hummers around the world to report their experiences. The result is the World Hum Map and Database [51]. He has accumulated over 7000 entries, with a particular concentration in the United States, the British Isles, and Western Europe. Western Australia and New Zealand were also hot spots. There were even reports from Iceland and Greenland. Not surprisingly, English-speaking countries dominated the database since the website was in English. There were no Hummers from Russia or China. Men and women were about equally affected and most were between the ages of 20 and 60 years. The most common self-reported symptoms were sleep disturbance (in nearly all), followed by fatigue, ear discomfort and irritability. Other symptoms were less frequent. Descriptions were remarkably variable but certain words kept coming up: motor, diesel engine, car or truck idling, airplane, refrigerator, industrial machine, and subwoofer. People were asked to try and match the frequency of their hum using an online tone generator. The majority estimated frequencies of between 20 and 100 Hertz. No one frequency dominated; about 5% were estimated to have been between 100 and 500 Hertz, while a few were judged to have been above 1000 Hertz. Nearly all reported hearing 'the Hum' in their homes, but it could be in different locations, upstairs, ground level, in the bedroom or other specific rooms. The sound was consistently loudest at night and not localized to either ear.

Being a hummer himself and the creator of the worldwide map and database, MacPherson was naturally interested in investigating the source. But his investigative techniques so far have been more along the lines of Peter Sellers' Inspector Clouseau than Sir Arthur Conan Doyle's Sherlock Holmes. In an article published in *The New Republic* in April 2016, reporter Colin Dickey described his visit to Gibsons to discuss 'the Hum' with MacPherson [30]. To get to this remote town, he took the Trans-Canada Highway west as far as it went, ending at Horseshoe Bay. From there he took a ferry across Howe Sound past sparsely inhabited islands before finally arriving. MacPherson told him about his personal experience with 'the Hum' and his efforts to develop his global database. He described his interest in Deming's article and the idea that 'the Hum' could result from VLF radio waves. Deming had suggested a simple set of experiments to test the hypothesis: make three boxes large enough for a human subject, one that blocked sound waves, one that blocked VLF and other electromagnetic waves, and a third control box that blocked neither [11, p 591]. MacPherson was surprised that no hummer had attempted to conduct the experiment so he crowdsourced a few hundred dollars and built one of the boxes – the box to block out VLF electromagnetic waves. Deming had suggested using the box with one-inch thick aluminum walls but this would have been very expensive and technically challenging so he looked for a substitute: "Then I went on with my research and discovered that mild steel, with a minimum thickness of 1.2 millimeters, would provide what they call, in the physics lingo, about ten skin depths. Each skin depth of mild steel attenuates the signal to about 30% of what the original signal strength would be. Ten skin depths essentially provides 100% coverage" [30, p 55]. So if a hummer heard the sound outside of the box and it disappeared inside the box it likely was due to VLF electromagnetic waves.

MacPherson took Dickey to see his steel box which he had constructed in a woodshed that was covered but not sealed. The welds of the box were thick and covered all seams since VLF waves can penetrate even the slightest crack. MacPherson noted, "If it were a different frequency than VLF, like something around microwave, or cell phone frequency, which some people suggest, then this would not have taken me off and on 3 years to build" [30, p 56]. Microwave and cell phone waves could be easily blocked with a thin layer of aluminum foil. He opened the hatch and showed Dickey the inside which was just big enough to cram in a human subject. He reassured Dickey that a box that size had enough oxygen for about 4 hours of breathing. Of course, Dickey's first question was – what happened when you got in the box? He was surprised to hear that MacPherson *had not gotten into the box*. He gave a variety of excuses for not doing the experiment including that it might not work in the open shed, the box was too big to fit through the door of his house, he would need a trailer to take it to someone's garage and that he didn't want it to be seen in public. Dickey offered to rent a U-Hall but MacPherson changed the subject preferring a theoretical discussion to performing the experiment. After a few weeks of hearing that MacPherson was going to conduct the experiment in front of him, Dickey realized that it was not going to happen. MacPherson provided further excuses: the new school year was beginning and he had no time for his "hobbies" and the experiment was not practical since even if positive, people cannot live in an airtight steel box all their life [30, p 57].

More recently, MacPherson decided to investigate 'the Hum' further on a visit to Russia. He wanted to know if the sound could be heard there, and whether the Russians had done experiments on it during the Cold War. If he could hear 'the Hum' in Russia, he planned to measure the frequency using an online tone generator to see if it was the same as in North America. He noted that the electric grid in Russia is at 50 Hertz while it is 60 Hertz in North America. If 'the Hum' had anything to do with the electrical grid, it should change frequency in Russia. He posted his experiences after returning from Russia on July 30, 2018 [51]. With regard to his efforts to learn what the Russians knew about 'the Hum,' he decided to visit the main library in St. Petersburg to look for relevant material as he had studied the Russian language. MacPherson provided the following explanation for failing to complete this task: he had not been allowed into the library by security as he had left his passport at his apartment. He could have easily returned with his passport, but he leaves it at that and never returned to the library [51]. On his fourth day in Russia, he heard 'the Hum' for the first time, although it was not as distinct as at home. He speculated that as St. Petersburg is heavily populated and noisy, the night-time window for hearing 'the Hum' was smaller than in rural Canada. His answer to the question of the frequency of the Russian hum, was stunning. "I'm sorry but I can't answer that accurately. I opened up the online tone generator several times, but I couldn't get a good match like I can here. I am quite confident that it is the same general range (i.e., low 50s Hz to mid-60s Hz)" [51].

So, after all this, what is the source of 'the Hum?' First, we have no doubt that most people are hearing *something* and those who get sick have *real symptoms*. But that does not mean that there is some villain out there traveling around the world secretly generating sounds that annoy and sicken people. In many instances, there may not even be an actual sound causing the problem. One thing that is clear from perusing the data, there is no single hum that everyone hears – a global hum. There are too many different descriptions, and the frequencies and loudness vary considerably, while the circumstances for hearing 'the Hum' vary even more. Could 'the Hum' simply represent tinnitus as has been suggested by many [52]. Ringing in the ears is extremely common in the general population and most people with this condition have normal hearing. We now know that tinnitus results from reverberating signals in brain auditory pathways and can occur even in people who are deaf. In fact, it often becomes worse if people with tinnitus begin to lose their hearing. Like 'the Hum,' tinnitus tends to be most bothersome at night when it is quiet. Background sounds such as a fan or music are helpful for masking both 'the Hum' and tinnitus. Glen MacPherson noticed that his hum could be briefly shut off by turning his head to the side or if he forcibly exhaled, features that can sometimes be seen with tinnitus. Another prominent feature shared by Hummers and tinnitus sufferers is that the more they focus on the sound, the more bothersome it becomes. Therapies for both conditions have focused on decreasing the person's focus on the sound using techniques such as cognitive behavioral and mindfulness therapy. But tinnitus persists in all locations and is typically described as a high-pitched ringing or buzzing sound, while 'the Hum' is usually described as low-pitched and is typically only heard indoors in the evening, often within a narrow time frame [53].

The body produces all sorts of sounds that can be bothersome. Many people can hear normal blood flow in arteries and veins that run close by the ear. Blood flow through arteries typically is pulsatile, timed with the heartbeat, but blood flow in veins can be heard as a continuous sound with a whooshing quality. A so-called venous hum is usually associated with hearing venous blood flow in the jugular vein and bulb located near the ear. The sound can be heard on one or both sides and in some people with large jugular bulbs, the sound can be quite bothersome. The sound varies in intensity depending on the volume and speed of the blood flow and is more noticeable in the quiet at night. However, this does not explain the restricted locations for hearing the sound described by most Hummers.

One way to explain frequent observations that 'the Hum' is just heard inside buildings is that sound is being generated within these structures, but scientists have looked for 'the Hum' using sophisticated recording devices and found no sound or infrasound in the buildings of Hummers. Further, resonant sounds generated within the structures' ductwork should shut off when the power is shut off. Could they be hearing electromagnetic waves? The ear has evolved to be sensitive to sounds, not electromagnetic waves. The eardrum and middle ear ossicles (bones in the inner ear that transmit sounds) are set into motion by sound waves but are insensitive to electromagnetic waves. Sound waves and electromagnetic waves are two different phenomena with completely different properties. Electromagnetic waves move much faster. That is why you see lightning well before you hear the thunder. Electromagnetic waves also contain much more energy than sound waves. For example, a cell phone puts out electromagnetic waves with about a watt of power per square meter, whereas routine sound waves that you hear have less than one-hundredth of a watt. If you could hear the electromagnetic waves from your cell phone it would be a very loud clacking and clattering sound, not a hum [54]. The notion that electromagnetic waves of any frequency could be the source of 'the Hum' is far-fetched. The one thing that Hummers generally agree on is that the sound is low frequency and localized to specific places whereas electromagnetic waves produce a perceived high-frequency sound in people with good high-frequency hearing and electromagnetic waves are pervasive in our society. Another possible explanation for 'the Hum' is that people hear sounds present in the everyday environment that everyone hears but for some reason they form a memory trace of the sound and cannot get it out of their mind. This type of mechanism has been proposed to explain some types of persistent tinnitus. A similar phenomenon can occur in other sensory systems, for example, a person suffers a painful injury and then has recurrences of the pain without any apparent reason.

Regardless of the source of 'the Hum,' there is little doubt that the mechanism of the symptoms is psychogenic in origin. There is no scientific evidence that 'the Hum' can cause physical damage to the brain or ears. Persistent noise exposure is known to trigger negative psychological reactions such as anxiety and depression. Just as with chronic pain, unpleasant noise can activate the limbic system, triggering fear and anger. Activation of the hypothalamic-pituitary-adrenal axis and autonomic nervous system triggers the fight or flight response. Most hummers realize that the noise they are "hearing" is not very loud yet their reaction is extreme. One hummer noted, "It's a kind of torture; sometimes, you just want to scream" [52]. Just the anticipation of the sound can cause them to become anxious. One hummer told a British reporter: "Last year it [the Hum] almost drove me to suicide, it completely drains energy, causing stress and loss of sleep. I have been on tranquilizers and have lost count of the number of nights I have spent holding my head in my hands, crying and crying" [11, p 576]. Just as with tinnitus, some hummers will learn to live with 'the Hum,' placing it in the back of their mind. It is still there but it no longer bothers them. This is the ultimate goal of treatments such as cognitive behavioral therapy and mindfulness therapy. Outbreaks of hum-induced illness such as those in Taos and Kokomo have many features in common with other outbreaks of mass psychogenic illness. An index case – the first person to exhibit symptoms, can serve as a template for others and the media then focuses attention on the sound and the symptoms that are expected. Once government agencies become involved in the search for the source of the sound, conspiracy theories begin to flourish. Negative expectations, hearing the sound and expecting to get sick, provide strong reinforce-ment for the outbreak. It is a classic setup for the nocebo effect. However, marketing may have changed the perception of 'the Hum.' For instance, while a few people in Taos still hear 'the Hum,' attention to it has died away and many of those who com-plained of serious symptoms have moved away. The Chamber of Commerce has even put a different spin on 'the Hum,' suggesting that if you come to Taos and hear it, it can be a sign of future good fortune and a long life. A California rock group even named their band *The Taos Hum.*

A similar phenomenon paralleling 'the Hum' has raised concerns since at least the early 1990s, in people living near high voltage power lines and power grids, have complained of an array of ailments paralleling those of hummers. These peo-ple attributed their ailments to the buzzing/droning sound. Some believe that this is the source of 'the Hum.' One concerned blogger warned the hummer community about the possible role of sound from powerlines, noting: "It is not just a Sound but is an Extremely Low Frequency/ELF (Radiation) Vibration in the Infrasonic range (–20 Hz) which is the same range as the human body's internal organs, which is why some of us actually FEEL the 'Hum' 'penetrating' & vibrating our gut, bladder, chest cavity, heart, brain, eyes, legs, feet. Yes, it is Slow Kill Torture!" [55, 56].

Wind Turbine Syndrome

With the recent advent of wind-to-energy technology, people living near wind farms have reported becoming sick from the noise created by the turning blades. Researchers studying the wind farm scare have demonstrated that the effects can be explained by mass psychology and expectation. In 2009, a panel of scientists found that a small number of people living near turbines experience health issues related to stress from the perception of noise, but not from the sound waves them-selves [57]. There is no evidence that sound below the threshold of human hearing has a negative effect on health. Human respiration and heart rate generate higher levels of sub-audible sound than those produced by rotating wind turbine blades! Many everyday sounds would occur at a higher level [58]. Despite consistent negative findings, wind farm opponents continue to blame an array of different health complaints on the sound [59].

One hotspot for Wind Turbine Syndrome opponents and protestors has been the rural eastern Australian town of Waubra in the State of Victoria, the site of one of the country's largest wind farms. Completed in July 2009, local residents began report-ing negative health effects attributed to the noise from the rotating turbines. These health concerns were highlighted nationally in 2011 with the broadcast of a docu-mentary by the Australian Broadcasting Corporation titled "Against the Wind." Among the complaints were high blood pressure, headaches, nausea, ear pressure, a tingling sensation, muscle spasms, strange sensations, lethargy, "ringing in the ears" and difficulty sleeping [60]. Local farmer Carl Stepnell and his wife Samantha were so disturbed by the noise that they decided to manage their local property dur-ing the day but never remained in their house overnight to avoid becoming unwell.

She said that her symptoms began within 6 months of the turbines going operational when she suffered from headaches and insomnia. At times she said it felt like she was "in a cabin of a plane. That's the only way I can explain it…the ear pressure and headaches - and the nausea…The longer I was around the turbines the worse I was feeling" [61].

Professor Simon Chapman from the School of Public Health at the University of Sydney observes that while some residents report feeling unwell and attribute their condition to the turbines, "there are also people who have them on their property, who live just as close or closer, who curiously don't say that it makes them ill" [61]. In explaining why some residents become ill while others do not, Professor Gary Wittert of the Adelaide University School of Medicine blames part of the problem on activists who incite fear. "If you whip up anxiety, people will generate many of these symptoms. There's fear of the unknown, there's activists creating concern among the population. We all get headaches from time to time. Now if someone comes along and tells you that your headaches are because there are wind turbines, now I know why I've got headaches," he said [61]. One study of Australians complaining about wind turbine noise and health problems found that the pattern of illness reports was suggestive of the role of social factors. It found that 65% of Australian wind farms – thirty-three in total – have never had a single complaint despite an estimated 21,633 residents living within five kilometers of the rotor blades. Furthermore, 73% of complaints in Australia were residents living near just six wind farms that had been targeted by wind turbine opposition groups. Most people (90%) "made their first complaint after 2009 when anti wind farm groups began to add health concerns to their wider opposition. In the preceding years, health or noise complaints were rare despite large and small-turbine wind farms having operated for many years" [62].

The psychogenic origin of Wind Turbine Syndrome is driven by expectation. Negative expectations increase the frequency and intensity of symptoms; positive expectations reduce them. Infrasound refers to low-frequency sound below the usual threshold of human hearing (typically below about 20 Hertz, although some people can hear sounds as low as 1.5 Hertz) [63]. The notion that infrasound can be dangerous to humans dates back to the early 1960s and the controversial work of the Russian-born French military scientist Vladimir Gavreau, who accidentally discovered that he and some of his colleagues were being made nauseous from a poorly mounted low-speed motor in the ventilation system of their building [64]. Mounted in the cavernous ducts of the several story building, the motor was causing nausea from the vibrating air column which formed a bizarre infrasonic amplifier. They realized that the vibration must have been very low in frequency since it did not register on any available sound detector. It was eventually shown to be in the range of 7 Hertz [65]. Subsequently, it has been a routine architectural procedure to search for such resonant cavities when remodeling older buildings.

As a military researcher, Gavreau immediately considered the potential implications of his discovery as an infrasonic military weapon. Could he produce a weapon that could cause symptoms but not be heard? He began to experiment with the building's ventilation system and noted that altering the spring tension on the shock mounts of the fan motor could change the frequency of the infrasonic resonances throughout the large building. Shutting the building's windows ameliorated the nauseating symptoms whereas opening the windows increased the symptoms. Gavreau's first experimental devises, organ pipe-like structures six feet in diameter and seventy-five-feet long, were designed to replicate the building's natural experiment. These devices were mounted to the outside of the building and the pipe output was driven by either a piston or compressed air. The resonant frequency of these pipes was in the range of three to seven Hertz, which was nicknamed the "range of death." Even though the investigators stood at a distance from the device and no sound was heard, symptoms came on rapidly within a few seconds of turning on the power. Gavreau reported that pressure waves gripped the entire body from all sides, followed by pain and pressure against the eyes and ears. Fortunately, one of the technicians was able to withstand the pain long enough to shut off the power supply. Gavreau and his fellow investigators were apparently ill for days after these preliminary tests with impaired vision and painful spasms in the chest and stomach. Presumably, the resonant body cavities absorbed the infrasound energy and would have been further damaged if the technician had not rapidly turned off the power. Gavreau had grossly misjudged the power released by the pipes [66].

To make a more compact and controllable infrasound generator, Gavreau had to lower the power and size. He began to test a variety of devices analogous to foghorns and police whistles. He developed a whistle, 1.3 meters in diameter, that probably produced a few watts per square meter in power at a frequency of about 40 Hertz that shook the walls of the laboratory complex. A large foghorn produced even more power at a higher frequency of about 150 Hertz. Gavreau, who had no background in acoustics and could not accurately measure the sound power or frequency, conducted studies that would be considered unethical by today's standards. Jörg Mühlhans, a psychoacoustic expert at the University of Vienna concluded, "I have no idea whatsoever where he got the numbers for sound pressure levels from, when he could not even measure infrasound at all" [66]. The key point that Gavreau failed to comprehend is that extremely high energy sound at any frequency can be harmful to humans. He was generating sound with several watts of power per square meter compared to the hundredths of a watt of power per square meter in commonly heard sounds including common low-frequency sounds. Gavreau concluded that high-energy infrasound might be used as a military weapon. Indeed, the French government experimented with "sound ray" weapons in the late 1960s but gave up on the project because of the impracticality of producing high powered sound weapons that were often more dangerous to the operators than the enemy. It is important to note that just because dangerous high-energy low-frequency sound can be produced, it does not mean that infrasound by nature is dangerous. An analogy is to assume that the explosion in a cap gun is dangerous because the explosion of a two-ton bomb is dangerous. Low-energy infrasounds are very common in everyday life and are generated by such varied sources as ocean waves and bedroom fans. Large animals like whales and elephants use infrasound to communicate. Some people complain that infrasound is annoying and can produce a wide range of symptoms from headaches and dizziness to anxiety and depression. Numerous articles in the print media along with testimonials from popular figures such as David Bowie and William Burroughs have heightened the public's fear of infrasound [66, p 4]. An infrasonic frequency between 5 and 9 Hertz was jokingly referred to as the "brown note" since it was said to immediately cause a human subject to defecate due to resonance in the colon. Fortunately, numerous attempts to hit the brown note with infrasound transmitted through the air, have been unsuccessful. A recent episode of the TV show MythBusters declared the 'brown note' to be a myth [67].

Wind turbines for generating clean energy have been around for decades, yet concerns about their health effects did not surface until the 1990s when it was first reported that they emitted infrasound. But unlike other potential mysterious environmental threats, it was easy to measure the power of infrasound emitted by modern-day wind turbines. They were found to be in the same low range – 20 to 40 decibels – as standing several meters from the ocean or a fan. This fact and numerous scientific studies showing no ill health effects of low-energy infrasound have not deterred advocates from trying to ban wind turbines. In 2010, then private citizen Donald Trump, provided his take on the controversy in an interview on *The Late Show with David Letterman*, criticizing how windfarms were not only "visually unattractive," they generate "a lot of noise." He told Letterman: "A lot of people that thought wind was great and [are] now saying, 'We have to live with these things for the rest of our lives." His alternative to wind was to mine more coal. Letterman provided the perfect response, "I'd rather see the windmills than the choking clouds of coal smoke" [68].

Into the debate stepped Dr. Nina Pierpoint, a pediatrician in Malone, New York, a campaigner against wind farms near her home. In 2009, Dr. Pierpoint self-published the book, *Wind Turbine Syndrome; A Report On a Natural Experiment* in which she described the case histories of 38 people who felt they developed symptoms from living near wind turbines [69]. She identified the people by placing ads in the areas of wind farms, asking for anyone who attributed their illness to wind turbines to contact her. She interviewed 23 of the 38 people over the phone; the other 15 were relatives of the 23, and their information was provided indirectly by the 23 contacts. As a control, she asked the 23 interviewees how they and their relative's health was prior to being exposed to wind turbines. Based on these case histories, Dr. Pierpont claimed that the turbines caused dizziness, tinnitus, headaches, loss of sleep and many other chronic symptoms. She became an instant celebrity with frequent interviews in the media and the darling of anti-wind groups internationally. In her book, Pierpont concluded that wind turbines generate infrasound that causes the illness. She noted that even though sound engineers play down the danger of low-frequency sound exposure, its ill effects have been documented in the laboratory and in the environment (by the likes of Professor Gavreau). Not surprisingly, the scientific community reacted negatively to the book, pointing out Dr. Pierpont's lack of background in acoustics or in conducting experimental studies and by her studying people who had already made up their minds that their symptoms were caused by exposure to wind turbines. Pierpont did not mention the extensive studies documenting the lack of effects of low power infrasound on human health [66].

A Social 'Illness'

Dr. Pierpont's book provided a spark for the already burgeoning international anti-wind turbine community; there are presently more than 2200 support groups globally [70]. Although present around the world, Wind Turbine Syndrome is conspicuously concentrated in English speaking countries. For example, Copenhagen probably has the largest concentration of wind turbines in Europe, yet Danes rarely develop the syndrome. Australia and New Zealand have been hotbeds for anti-wind turbine groups and demonstrations, significantly hampering the implementation of this much-needed clean energy source. A small number of wind farms that have been targeted by opposition groups have the most symptomatic patients. Seventy-five percent of cases were concentrated in six wind farms in Australia. In 2017, Simon Chapman observed: "I've counted 247 different diseases and symptoms in humans and animals attributed by opponents to wind farms. These include lung cancer, skin cancer, hemorrhoids, gaining and losing weight and my favorite, disoriented echidnas [a type of anteater]. But most are classic symptoms of anxiety: things that can happen to you when you are very worried." Chapman attributes the symptoms to the nocebo effect. "When some people are exposed to frightening information about agents or exposures, expectancy effects just as powerful as placebo effects can operate to make people feel sick with worry or anxiety. Twenty-five scientific reviews since 2003 have concluded that there is very poor evidence for any claim that wind turbines are the direct cause of any disease. Rather, a herd of uncontested elephants in the room point unavoidably to a conclusion that 'Wind Turbine Syndrome' is a communicated disease: you catch it by hearing about it and then worrying" [71]. In other words, it is a type of mass psychogenic illness.

Another mechanism for developing symptoms of Wind Turbine Syndrome is a heightened focus on symptoms that nearly everyone experiences. Normal, healthy people commonly exhibit headaches, dizziness, fatigue, difficulty concentrating and insomnia [58]. If people are worried about symptoms that might result from some environmental agent, they are more likely to notice and misattribute their own routine symptoms to something in the environment. A Canadian study analyzed symptoms reported by people living in the vicinity of wind turbines and found that the prevalence of reported complaints was the same as the prevalence of symptoms in the general population [58, p 3]. They concluded that people were misattributing their everyday symptoms to wind turbines and not developing a new sickness. When they think they hear the wind turbine noise, it signifies exposure to a perceived environmental threat, which provokes anxiety and a heightened focus on body sensations. Of course, anxiety itself can activate the adrenal gland and stimulate the nervous system, triggering symptoms of the fight or flight response. Interestingly, people tend to be bothered more by wind turbine sound if they can see the turbines. Presumably, seeing the blades reinforces the perceived threat. This, in combination with the sound, heightens the anxiety and worry, magnifying health fears.

If negative expectations can make you sick, then it should be possible to make you better with positive expectations. Researchers at the University of Auckland in New Zealand led by Health Psychology Professor Keith Petrie conducted experiments that showed this was the case [72]. They recruited 60 students (39 women and 21 men) and randomly assigned half to positive and half to negative expectation groups. Subjects were told that the purpose of the study was to investigate the effect of sound below the frequency of normal hearing on their physical sensations and mood. The sound exposure was conducted in a specially built sound room in the School of Engineering. Questionnaires were used to assess 24 common symptoms like headaches and fatigue, and the extent to which they felt 12 positive mood items (cheerful, relaxed, and so on), and 12 negative mood items (anxious, distressed, etc.). Symptoms and mood were assessed on a 7-point scale from 0 (not at all) to 6 (extreme). After baseline assessment, participants viewed one of two 5 ½ minute videos that contained health information about wind turbines readily available on the internet. The negative video included several recent TV programs suggesting that wind turbine sound, particularly infrasound, could pose health risks while the positive video provided an opposite point of view indicating that wind turbine sound contained infrasound, subaudible sound created by natural phenomena such as ocean waves and wind, which may have positive effects and therapeutic benefits on health. Participants were then exposed to wind farm sound that had been recorded 1 kilometer from a wind farm for two 7-minute listening sessions. They were told that they were listening to recorded wind farm sound and that it contained infrasound and audible sound. Symptom and mood questionnaires were completed during each exposure session. During exposure to the wind farm sound, symptoms and mood were strongly influenced by the type of expectations. Participants who had viewed the negative videos experienced a significant *increase* in symptoms and a significant deterioration in mood, while participants who viewed the positive videos reported a significant *decrease* in symptoms and a significant improvement in mood. The authors concluded that if expectations about wind farm sound, particularly infrasound, are framed in more neutral or even positive ways, people living near wind farms would be less likely to feel sick.

The same investigators then conducted a similar study on another group of 60 students but instead of assessing physical symptoms they assessed annoyance to wind farm noise after watching the same negative and positive videos [73]. Annoyance with environmental noise is pervasive in modern society. The researchers pointed out that although noise annoyance is not in itself a disease or health state, hypersensitivity to noise produces psychological stress that can lead to ill-health. Participants rated sensitivity to sound at baseline on a 4-point scale from 1 (not at all sensitive) to 4 (extremely sound sensitive). To assess the experience during the wind farm sound exposure sessions, subjects were asked if they found the sound exposure unpleasant, annoying, and irritating, on a 7-point scale from 0 (not at all) to 6 (extremely). For each exposure session, an annoyance score was calculated based on the combined scores of the three annoyance items. Participants who watched the positive videos were significantly less annoyed by the wind farm noise than participants who watched the negative videos. They concluded that negative information about sound can trigger annoyance particularly in people who are sound sensitive, and it may be possible to reduce sound annoyance even in people who are noise sensitive by providing a positive message about the sound.

Field studies have also found that annoyance with wind farm noise is highly dependent on people's perception of health risks and the context of the noise exposure [58]. Studies in Sweden and the Netherlands found that only about 25% of people living near wind farms were annoyed by the noise with only about 6% very annoyed. By contrast, about 60% of people in New Zealand living near wind farms complained of noise annoyance. These findings correlate with the generally positive media reports on wind farms in Sweden and the Netherlands and more negative reports in New Zealand particularly around the time when the high rate of noise annoyance was identified. Field studies consistently show that psychological and social factors are more important in annoyance to wind farm noise than the actual level of noise exposure. Studies in the Netherlands found that people who benefited economically from wind farms either with monthly stipends or partial ownership were much less likely to be annoyed by the noise than those without an economic interest. People with an economic interest in wind farms had the same awareness and sensitivity to sound as those without an economic interest but they had a different attitude toward the noise. Seeing and hearing wind turbines did not seem to bother them.

These findings on 'the Hum' and Wind Turbine Syndrome are directly relevant to the events in Cuba. Once rumors began to circulate that mysterious sounds were being generated by a sonic device, a self-fulfilling prophecy was created. Embassy staff began to redefine a variety of naturally occurring background noises – particularly crickets and cicadas, as being harmful to their health and thus generating significant anxiety. As a result, a nocebo pattern began to take shape. Add to this an array of ever-present symptoms that ordinarily would have been dismissed as normal aches and pain. The appearance of these complaints suddenly took on a new significance and were widely viewed as resulting from a sonic attack. Further reinforcing this new perspective were pronouncements by the State Department which doubled down on the attack claims, media stories, and studies appearing in one of the world's most prominent science publications, the *Journal of the American Medical Association*. Yet, in spite of all these factors adding to the picture that a real attack had taken place, the evidence to support those claims was not there.

References

1. Sagan C. Cosmos. London: Macdonald Futura; 1981.
2. Mystery humming noise is giving England residents sleepless nights. Herald Express (Torbay). 19 Aug 2014.
3. Gruber K. Giraffes spend their evening humming to each other. New Scientist Daily Newsletter. 17 Sept 2015.
4. Jamieson S. Zoo's neighbours claim noise from giraffe house is making them ill. The Daily Telegraph (London). 22 Feb 2016.
5. Baotic A, Sicks F, Stöger A. Nocturnal humming vocalizations: adding a piece to the puzzle of giraffe vocal communication. BMC Research Notes. 2015;8(8):425. (September 9).
6. Stallard B. The sound of giraffes? Night humming is key. Nature World News. 19 Sept 2015.
7. Bevan T. Giraffes humming could be disturbing zoo neighbours and keeping them awake. The Daily Mirror (London). 2 Oct 2015.

8. Nodal JH. Comments and answers. The hummadruz, in City news notes and queries reprinted from the Manchester City News. Manchester: City News Office. 29 Jun 1878.
9. Many Britons go sleepless from 'big hum,' Springfield Union (MA). 17 Jun 1960. p. 7.
10. Jangles Nerves: Britions are bothered by mysterious hum. Greensboro Daily News (NC). 25 Apr 1960. p. 1.
11. Deming D. The hum: an anomalous sound heard around the world. J Sci Explor. 2004;18(4):571–95. See p. 573.
12. McQuillan R. Torture of the twilight zone: Largs hum sufferer Georgie Hyslop turns detective in bid to solve mystery. The Herald (Glasgow, Scotland). 28 Sept 2001.
13. Barton B. What's that noise? it's a constant, irritating hum that makes life miserable for all who hear it – but nobody knows what it is. The Guardian. 18 Oct 2001.
14. Alexander J. Have you heard 'the hum?' BBC News. 19 May 2009.
15. McQuillan R, Martin L. Mystery of the Largs hum drones on; msp calls for executive investigation into low-frequency noise that causes sickness and pain. The Herald (Glasgow). 26 Jan 2001. p. 3.
16. Hum makes people sick. The Mirror (London). 26 Jan 2001. p. 2.
17. McQuillan R. Mystery hum forces couple out of home; call for low frequency noise phenomenon to be investigated by Holyrood committee. The Herald (Glasgow). 19 Mar 2001. p. 9.
18. Sieveking P. Hum rattles teeth across Scotland droning on, The Sunday Telegraph (London). 6 May 2001. p. 31.
19. Tweedie N. So can you hear the hum?: Neil Tweedie listens for the mysterious rumbling that's tormenting a whole village, The Daily Telegraph (London). 17 Jun 2011. p. 23.
20. McBeth J. Will this hum ever buzz off? Daily Mail (London). 4 Jul 2011. p. 15.
21. Butterworth A. Help, our village is haunted...by a mysterious hum. The Daily Mail (London) 19 Oct 2018. p. 13.
22. Mysterious 'Bristol hum' prompts official inquiry. Wichita Eagle (KS). 18 Mar 1980. p. 10.
23. Lambert P, Haederle M. Hmmmmmmmmmmmm...? The riddle of the sands of Taos, New Mexico, is a harbinger: what on earth is making that unearthly sound? People. 1998;38:61.
24. Radford B. What is the Taos hum? Live Science. 20 Feb 2014.
25. Taos hum interm reports. https://sites.google.com/site/gridsick/taos-hum-interim-reports. Accessed 4 Oct 2019.
26. Cowan JP. The results of hum studies in the United States, Ninth International Congress on Noise as a Public Health Problem. Foxwoods; 2008.
27. Baker D. Next Toas study to focus on those who hear hum. Denver Post. 25 Aug 1993.
28. Gore-Langton R. What is the truth behind spooky Bristol hum? The Express (London). 25 Feb 2016. p. 13.
29. Brightmore J. The Bristol hum. https://jamiebrightmore.com/other/the-bristol-hum/. Accessed 23 May 2019.
30. Dickey C. A maddening sound. Is the hum, a mysterious noise heard around the world, science or mass delusion? The New Republic. 8 Apr 2016, pp.1–16.
31. Spilman R. The hum heard round the world – From Sausalito to Seattle to Southhampton, mating midshipmen fish keeping the neighbors awake. The Old Salt Blog. 25 Oct 2013. http://www.oldsaltblog.com/2013/10/the-hum-heard-round-the-world-from-sausalito-to-seattle-to-south-hampton-mating-midshipmen-fish-keeping-the-neighbors-awake/. Accessed 23 Apr 2019.
32. Novak C. Investigation of the Windsor hum. University of Windsor. Final Report. Government of Canada, Office of Global Affairs. 5 May 2014. http://www.international.gc.ca/department-ministere/windsor_hum_results-bourdonnement_windsor_resultats.aspx?lang=eng. Accessed 14 Aug 2019.
33. Storm from Windsor fans over Zug Island. Detroit Times. 16 Jan 1959. p. 4.
34. Mele C. There's a persistent hum in this Canadian city, and no one knows why. The New York Times. 19 Feb 2018.
35. Results of study on Windsor hum released. Targeted News Service (Washington, DC). 23 May 2014.

36. Vieira P. Canadian study says 'Windsor hum' is for real; mysterious noise likely comes from island on Michigan side of Detroit River, Canada says. The Wall Street Journal Online 23 May 2014.
37. Results of UWindsor hum research released. University of Windsor Daily News. 26 May 2014. http://www.uwindsor.ca/dailynews/music/2014-05-25/results-uwindsor-hum-research-released. Accessed 10 Aug 2019.
38. Schmidt D. Mayor seeks sit-down with U.S. steel to talk about Windsor hum. Windsor Star. 21 Jul 2016.
39. Fountain JW. Hum haunts Indiana city; it's source is a mystery. The New York Times. 23 Jun 2002.
40. Huppke R. Strange doings abuzz in Kokomo – many claim illness from mystery noise. Bergen County Record (NJ). 13 Jun 2002.
41. Kozarovich LH. Residents complain of illness, cite factory hum. Kokomo Tribune (IN). 17 Jul 2001.
42. Falda W. Bad vibrations in Kokomo lead to illness and even death, some say; others skeptical. South Bend Tribune (IN). 25 Aug 2002.
43. Huppke RW. In Indiana city, it's not hum, sweet hum; mystery noise fuels Kokomo complaints. The Washington Post. 9 Jun 2002; Sect. pA:17;
44. Stuteville G. Kokomo is abuzz over real humdinger. Indianapolis Star (IN). 19 Feb 2002.
45. Kozarovich LH. Residents ask for help. Kokomo Tribune. 10 Feb 2002.
46. Stedman L. City wants to muffle 'Kokomo hum. Courier-Journal (Louisville, KY). 29 Dec 2003.
47. Lewis K. Expert says hum is not a sound. Kokomo Tribune (IN). 3 Jun 2004.
48. The Kokomo hummers. The Fortean Times (London). 2011;162:26–7(April).
49. Cowan JP. The Kokomo hum investigation. Acentech Project No. 615411. Cambridge: Acentech Incorporated; 2002.
50. Libaw O. Complaints surround mysterious 'Kokomo hum.' ABC News (NY). 13 Feb 2002.
51. MacPherson G. https://hummap.wordpress.com/. Accessed 2 May 2019.
52. Lallanilla M. Mysterious hum driving people crazy around the world. ABC News (NY). 26 Jul 2016.
53. Otoacoustic emissions are sounds that arise in the ear canal when the ear drum receives vibrations transmitted backwards from the cochlea through the middle ear during the process of normal hearing. The sound which is typically in the speech range of 1–4,000 Hertz, can be heard by some people although it is very soft. Most people learn to ignore the sound just as you learn to ignore the sensation of your backside against a chair when sitting for some time. See: Kemp D. Otoacoustic emissions, their origin in cochlear function, and use. Br Med Bull. 2002;63(1):223–41.
54. Elder JA, Chou CK. Auditory response to pulsed radiofrequency energy. Bioelectromagnetics Suppl 6 (2002): S162–73. Studies show that even though the middle ear conduction system is completely insensitive to electromagnetic waves, some people with good high frequency hearing can detect electromagnetic waves as weak high frequency sound (like electrical static). This implies that some electromagnetic waves can create an acoustic vibration in the cochlea (the part of the ear that receives sounds in the form of vibrations) that gets detected as high-frequency sound. Electrical potentials inside the cochlea evoked by electromagnetic pulses have been recorded and they look just like potentials evoked by sound waves. Interestingly, the sound heard is independent of the frequency of the electromagnetic waves but rather is dependent on the dimensions of the person's head. Somehow, the electromagnetic wave energy is absorbed by the head and this energy is transformed into tiny pressure waves that directly stimulate the base of the cochlea just as high frequency sound does. The delicate hair cells in the cochlea are sensitive to molecular size displacements of the cochlear fluid.

55. Moore J. Mysterious ELF sound agonizes New Mexico; spreads across the nation. The Phoenix Foundation Newsletter http://amasci.com/hum/newshum.txt. Accessed 15 Jan 2018.
56. Yes to powergrid, blog posting to the 'noise help' website. https://www.noisehelp.com/humming-sound.html. Accessed 4 Nov 2018.
57. Colby WD, Dobie R, Leventhall G, Lipscomb D, McCunney R, Seilo M, et al. Wind turbine sound and health effects: an expert panel. Report prepared for American Wind Energy Association and Canadian Wind Energy Association. 2009.
58. Crichton F, Chapman S, Cundy T, Petrie KJ. The link between health complaints and wind turbines: support for the nocebo expectations hypothesis. Front Public Health. 2014;2(220):1–8. https://doi.org/10.3389/fpubh.2014.00220.
59. Chapman S. Wind turbine syndrome: a communicated disease, paper presented to Royal Society of NSW Symposium on The Future of Rationality in a Post-Truth World, Government House (Sydney, Australia). 29 Nov 2017. p. 3.
60. Tran D. Can wind turbines make you sick? Debate divides tiny Victorian town of Waubra. Australian Broadcasting Corporation (Sydney). 24 Mar 2017.
61. Fowler A, O'Brien K. Against the wind. Australian broadcasting corporation (Sydney). Airing 25 Jul 2011.
62. Chapman S, St George A, Waller K, Cakic V. The pattern of complaints about Australian wind farms does not match the establishment and distribution of turbines: support for the psychogenic, 'communicated disease' hypothesis. PLoS One. 2013;8(10):c76584. https://doi.org/10.1371/journal.pone.0076584. See p. 1.
63. Leventhall G. What is ultrasound? Prog Biophys Mol Bio. 2007;93:130–7.
64. Gavreau V. Infrasound Science Journal 1968;4:33–37.
65. Vassilatos G. Deadly sound: Vladimir Gavreau. Borderlands. 14 Sept 2011.
66. Jaeki P. Why people believe low-frequency sound is dangerous. The Atlantic. 19 Jun 2017. p. 3.
67. Brown Note, Accessed online at http://www.discovery.com/tv-shows/mythbusters/mythbusters-database/brown-note/.
68. DonaldTrumponDavidLetterman–2010.https://www.youtube.com/watch?v=mwxqgo9XO5c. Accessed 20 Nov 2019.
69. Pierpont N. Wind turbine syndrome. Santa Fe (NM): K-selected Books; 2009.
70. Links to over 2200 International Anti-Wind Groups. https://quixoteslaststand.com/worldwide-anti-wind-groups/. Accessed 23 Sept 2019.
71. Chapman S. How to catch 'wind turbine syndrome': by hearing about it and worrying. The Guardian. 28 Nov 2017.
72. Crichton F, Dodd G, Schmid G, Gamble G, Cundy T, Petrie KJ. The power of positive and negative expectations to influence reported symptoms and mood during exposure to wind farm sound. Health Psychol. 2014;33(12):1588–92.
73. Crichton F, Dodd G, Schmid G, Petrie KJ. Framing sound: using expectations to reduce environmental noise annoyance. Environ Res. 2015;142:609–14.

Phantom Assailants: Mad Gassers, Phantom Slashers, and Other Believed-in Imaginings

8

Of all the passions, fear weakens judgment most.

–Jean Francois Paul de Gondi de Retz [1]

Within the annals of the social sciences, there is an entire genre of cases that closely parallel the Cuban 'sonic attack' affair: the literature on phantom assailants. *Hundreds* of similar cases have been recorded over the centuries. Only the form changes to reflect current fears. When we include cases attributed to demons and witches during the Middle Ages – and in many parts of Africa, Asia, and South America today, the number of episodes easily numbers in the thousands. In this chapter, we will describe some of the more prominent outbreaks. Episodes are divided between assailants who are believed to make people sick and those that are thought to physically accost their victims. All of these episodes can be considered social delusions, but only *some* involve psychogenic illness. Like all social panics, they reflect prevailing anxieties and are limited only by plausibility. At their core lies the rapid, spontaneous spread of false beliefs. The old English proverb, "Talk of the devil and he is bound to appear," was never more apropos than to the phenomenon of phantom assailants as it underscores the power of fear and expectation [2]. There is a similar saying from Japan: "Talk of a man and his shadow will show up" [2]. Outbreaks are driven by the fallibility of human perception and memory reconstruction. Just how easy it is for humans to fool themselves is evidenced in the case of the Russian Zond IV moon probe which unexpectedly fell back to earth on the night of March 3, 1968, creating a series of spectacular 'meteors' streaking across the eastern US from Pennsylvania to Kentucky. One eyewitness told Air Force officers that he saw what appeared to be "square-shaped windows" and a metallic fuselage with a "riveted-together look." He continued: "I toyed with the idea that it even slowed down somewhat, for how else could we observe so much detail in a mere flash across the sky?" The three witnesses agreed that they had observed "a craft from Outer Space" [3]. Another classic example is the case of the Rotterdam panda. In 1978, a panda escaped from a zoo in Holland's second largest city, prompting

© Springer Nature Switzerland AG 2020
R. W. Baloh, R. E. Bartholomew, *Havana Syndrome*,
https://doi.org/10.1007/978-3-030-40746-9_8

hundreds of panda sightings across the area in the following days. The panda was eventually found dead near train tracks not far from the zoo. It was soon evident that the animal had been killed shortly after it had gotten loose [4].

Phantom assailant outbreaks often coincide with periods of perceived danger and reflect a specific threat. The mass media commonly play a key role in the creation, maintenance, and eventual extinguishment of these episodes, initially presenting stories that treat the danger as real, while near the end of the outbreak, reporting skeptical accounts which contribute to its decline. Understanding the social and cultural context of cases is vital. For instance, during the Scandinavian 'ghost rocket' scare of 1946, authorities were inundated with hundreds of sightings of rockets that were believed to have been test-fired by Russia as a form of intimidation. The sightings occurred amidst the political uncertainty following the close of the Second World War. While sensational press coverage fueled the episode, a key factor was the poor state of relations between the Soviet Union and northern Europe. Sweden, Norway, and Finland have a long history of border disputes and invasion fears with the former Soviet state and before that, Russia, dating back to the nineteenth century. It was within this context of fear and suspicion that Scandinavians began to redefine astronomical and meteorological events as ghost-rocket related [5, 6]. More recently, social panics involving psychogenic symptoms have been more frequent in Western countries and take the form of pseudo-terror attacks. On September 29, 2001, innocuous fumes from oil-based paints were sent wafting through the air at Canyon Creek Middle School in Washington State, triggering a mass casualty event. The social climate in America at the time was a huge factor in the outbreak because the incident happened shortly after the September 11 terrorist attacks on the United States. Hence, the smell was interpreted as a terrorist event. As a result, 16 students were rushed to hospital after experiencing dizziness, fainting and "anxiety attacks" [7].

The first category of phantom assailants involves imagined attacks that feature mass psychogenic illness. Contemporary episodes commonly have a terror-related theme and typically occur amid actual terrorism incidents and media reports which highlight the threat. Like most cases of psychogenic illness, they often begin with a trigger such as a strange smell, a sound or something suspicious-looking that makes people suspect that they are in harm's way. Sometimes, unbeknownst to the rest of the group, the first person to exhibit symptoms may have an organic illness. In school outbreaks, young girls seem to be particularly vulnerable but anyone including male students and staff can be affected and extreme anxiety can spread by sight, word of mouth, and media. A strange odor is the most common trigger of mass psychogenic illness. It is critically important to distinguish between psychogenic and organic causes for symptoms early in the process since victims of mass toxic exposure may require decontamination, antidotes and extensive medical testing whereas victims of mass psychogenic illness need reassurance and a plausible explanation for their symptoms.

In many developing countries where outbreaks are dominated by the appearance of motor symptoms instead of a mysterious odor, long-term stress is the cause, with the content of cases colored by local folklore. A sample of African, Asian, and South

American cases from 2018 alone, reveals dozens of separate outbreaks during the year, highlighting the extent of the problem. Most of these episodes were fueled by the unshakable belief in the existence of evil spirits, and anxiety generated by rumors that sorcerers and witchdoctors are active in their school, placing curses on students. The pattern in many of these cases involves reports of demonic possession and convulsions as students enter trance states. Sometimes the threat is more diffuse, such as sightings of ghosts. The Philippines were a hotbed for 'attacks' during the year' [8–14]. One of the largest occurred in Cebu during June. A Manila newspaper reported on the case with the headline, "Evil spirits 'Possess' 46 Students in Ronda, Argao."

CEBU, Philippines – Classes were suspended yesterday in two national high schools in Ronda and Argao towns after 46 students were "possessed" by evil spirits.

The students of Ronda National High School were preparing to participate in the national earthquake drill around 10 a.m. when 26 of them started to show signs of "evil possession," prompting the Bureau of Fire Protection personnel to cancel the activity.

The school officials also decided to suspend classes while the affected students were immediately rushed to the rural health unit and the church.

… In Argao, an adjacent town in the southeast of Ronda, another school experienced a similar phenomenon yesterday afternoon.

At least 20 students of Colawin National High School were also said to have been "possessed" by evil spirits prompting school officials to also suspend classes.

One of the students (name withheld) said her classmate suddenly cried after she allegedly saw a lady in the comfort room of their classroom around 1 p.m. yesterday. [15]

In affirming the reality of demons in the outbreak, a local Catholic priest, Father Ric Reyes, said that the Church recognizes the belief in the invisible world of demons that is acknowledged during mass [15].

During February, a Satanism scare erupted at a school in Zimbabwe when sorcery paraphernalia was found on the grounds, after which several Grade 7 students felt dizzy and collapsed, believing they had been cursed. The school was closed for 2 weeks after students were refusing to enter the premises until the 'curse' was lifted. A *tsikamutanda* (witch-hunter) was eventually summoned [16]. The following month, a group of Catholic schoolgirls in the Mid-lands province started screaming, fainting and experienced convulsions; they were believed to have been possessed by demons [17]. The presence of evil spirits were attributed to separate similar attacks in Uganda in September and October [18, 19]. The fear of ghosts was blamed for outbreaks in Ghana, [20] Malaysia, [21] and India, [22] while children playing with a Ouija board triggered an event among 30 students in Peru during September which inlcuded screaming, convulsions and demonic possession [23].

Mad Gassers

Two seemingly bizarre episodes of mass psychogenic illness involving phantom assailants were triggered by strange odors in small towns in Virginia and Illinois during the first half of the twentieth century. However, when one begins to examine the context of these cases, it becomes clear that they were products of their times and reflected popular fears. To understand these episodes, one must consider the setting in which they occurred. From the time the Germans released chlorine gas in Ypres, Belgium on April 22, 1915, poison gas was the most feared weapon of mass destruction in the world. More than 5000 Allied soldiers were killed and 10,000 were injured at Ypres and by the end of the war, at least 90,000 soldiers were killed and over a million injured by a variety of poison gasses that were used by both sides. Who can forget the famous painting, *Gassed*, by the American artist John Singer Sargent, showing a line of soldiers blinded by mustard gas, each with his hand on the soldier in front being led along a road to receive treatment. Along the side of the road, hundreds of injured soldiers awaited help. In the summer of 1918, the 62-year-old Sargent traveled to France and Belgium as an official war artist for Britain. The painting was based on a scene he had witnessed at Le-Bac-du Sud on the Arras-Doullens Road. After the war, the fear of poison gas was indelibly etched into the American psyche. It seemed that the use of poison gas was inevitable as preparations for poison gas defense became routine in countries around the world. The mass media regularly ran stories about the dangers of future gas attacks and how to prepare for them. This historical backdrop was fertile soil for two separate 'mad gasser' panics [24–26].

The Mad Gasser of Virginia

From December 1933 to February 1934 several small towns in rural central Virginia were fear-stricken by newspaper and radio reports of someone sneaking about in the night releasing poison gas that caused residents to fall ill. It seemed as though the 'mad gasser' could come and go at will without being detected despite a concerted effort by local police who were frustrated because they could not find any objective evidence of a gas or perpetrator. Near the end of the episode, police grew concerned that innocent people may be harmed as armed residents began patrolling roads at night with loaded guns. The 'attacks' occurred in two waves, originating in Botetourt County, and later in adjacent Roanoke County.

The first gas attack occurred at the farmhouse of Cal Huffman in Haymakertown, a tiny village with about 30 people, a few days before Christmas 1933. At around 10 p.m. on December 22, Mrs. Huffman reported smelling a gas-like odor causing her to feel dizzy and nauseous. She went to bed but her husband stayed up to investigate. About half an hour later he also thought he smelled gas and he called the police who did not arrive until after midnight. O. D. Lemon, an officer who was well known locally for his crime-solving skills, responded and searched the house and property. He found nothing and left by 1 am. Shortly after, a third "gas attack" took place at the Huffman residence involving all six children who became ill; the most severely affected was Alice their 20-year-old daughter who fainted. A local doctor, S. F. Driver was called to the house and upon finding Alice unconscious, administered "artificial respiration" in order to "resuscitate" her. While sounding dramatic, in reality, it appears that she had simply fainted and was said to have completely recovered within a few hours, only to have later relapsed, which Dr. Driver attributed to "nerves." After this third 'attack,' Mr. Huffman said he *may* have seen a man running away [27]. The series of incidents on the night of the 22nd and the early morning hours of the 23rd, were reported on in sensational fashion in the *Roanoke Times* on Christmas Eve. "Gas 'Attack' on Family is Probed. Fumes at Night Fell Girl and Make Others Ill at Haymakertown Home..." The county coroner, Dr. W. N. Breckinridge speculated that the gas may have been "chicken gas" often used by chicken thieves to briefly knock out chickens while they were being snatched.

News of the 'attacks' spread by word of mouth, on the radio and in the local press, priming the community to be on the lookout for the gasser. Of significance here is the way in which the story was reported in the newspaper. The next article on the affair appeared in the *Roanoke Times* on December 27, treating the gasser attacks as factual, with the accompanying headline: "Gas Attacks on Homes Continue." The story detailed a separate incident, involving Mr. and Mrs. Clarence Hall of Cloverdale. After returning home from church with their three children, the Halls noted an odor that they described as leaving a sickeningly sweet taste in their mouths. At first, Mr. Hall thought fumes were coming from the stove but when they became sick, he called authorities. Their symptoms included severe nausea, weakness and some burning of the eyes. Dr. Breckinridge came to the house and suggested that the odor smelled something like formaldehyde but he wasn't sure. The women left the house and went to stay with nearby relatives while the men stayed in the woods armed with guns waiting for the gasser [28]. Relatives driving by the house the next night thought they caught a glimpse of someone with a flashlight near the Hall's house but were afraid to stop. The 'gasser' struck again on the 27th at Troutville as a local welder named A.L. Kelly said he was attacked at about 10 p.m. while upstairs in his house. Strangely, none of the other occupants of the house were affected [29]. Officer Lemon noted that the only evidence he was able to uncover was the print of what appeared to a woman's high-heel shoe found under the window where the gas was likely sprayed into the Huffman's house. He began looking for a man with a female accomplice [30].

After this initial flurry of attacks, there was a brief reprieve and people began to settle down but this was short-lived and the attacks recurred with increasing frequency. On January 11, the gasser attacked the house of Homer Hylton at Howell's Mill a few miles from the county seat of Fincastle. The Hyltons slept upstairs and the wife of a traveling salesman, Mrs. Moore slept downstairs. Mrs. Moore thought she heard whispering in the yard followed by a rustling of a shade next to a window. She then smelled gas and felt numb all over. She grabbed her baby and ran from the house screaming. The Hyltons did not notice any odors and were not sick, but Mr. Hylton stood guard with a shotgun outside the home for the rest of the night. With this attack, word rapidly spread throughout Botetourt County and the number of reported attacks rapidly escalated. After an attack at the home of G. D. Kinzie in Troutville, Dr. Driver concluded that potentially lethal chlorine gas was used despite the minor symptoms suffered by the inhabitants. In another incident, Officer Lemon spotted another footprint of a woman's high-heel shoe near where a car had been parked along the road. But police were baffled by the lack of concrete evidence of poison gas or the method that the gas was delivered. Even more confounding was the motive for the attacks [31].

The fear of a crazed gasser on the loose reached a fever peak in late January after several more houses were attacked, but without any trace of the assailant. Families stayed together while the menfolk patrolled the roads late in the evening or sat on their doorsteps with loaded guns. After one of the gas attacks, police were called immediately; they responded on the only two roads leading into the property sure that they had trapped the culprit, but he had eluded them again. On January 28 the house of Ed Stanley near Colon Siding was attacked and Mrs. Stanley suffered nausea along with a suffocating sensation and had to be carried from the house. The next morning, she and a houseguest were still groggy and unwell the next day but the doctor attributed the symptoms to sedatives and "nerves." Frank Guy, who worked for the family, rushed from the house and fired his shotgun at what appeared to be four men running near the woods. After another 'attack,' the son of a farmer opened fire at what appeared to be a man running in a field. Alerted by the barking of a guard dog, a man jumped out of bed, grabbed his shotgun, charged across a field and began shooting at what appeared to be a man creeping near a ditch. This was not a community to be out walking about! [32] Alarmed by the escalating events, the following day, the county Board of Supervisors offer a $500 reward for the apprehension and conviction of those responsible [33].

At this same time, some local officials were beginning to publicly express skepticism over the gasser's existence as some residents were viewing "the whole gassing case is a mere hoax, or figment of imagination of reported victims" [34]. During a meeting of the Board of Supervisors, Dr. Driver told his colleagues that while he believed the gasser was real, that some cases appeared to have been false alarms. For instance, it was revealed that at the home of one of the 'attacks,' the 'gas' was traced to a coal stove [35]. Sheriff L.T. Mundy perhaps best typified the mood. While declaring himself a "doubting Thomas" until gassed himself, his wife was stuffing keyholes to thwart the gasser [36]. As many began to suspect a hoax, the gasser scare faded in Botetourt County and moved to neighboring Roanoke County. On February 3, three people were sickened by the smell of gas in their house just outside of Vinton shortly after returning home. A local deputy Sheriff thought he could smell tear gas in the air when he arrived [37, 38]. A few days later, a Mrs. A. H. Milan and her daughter, Josephine noticed a funny smell coming from the door. Mrs. Milan had been sick and told her daughter that she felt worse. Then Josephine became dizzy [39]. Mrs. Milan spent the night in the hospital as a precaution [40].

Over the following two nights, the Roanoke policed received 12 further gasser calls, only to be frustrated by the lack of objective evidence. One of the callers who reported an attack, J. F. Clay, worked at the city health department. Mr. Clay, his wife, and two children were sitting in the front room when they noticed a strange odor. He and one of the children began to feel dizzy but when police detectives arrived, they could not detect any evidence of noxious fumes. Most of the calls were residents complaining of vague fumes but not falling sick. One report was triggered by a maid who over-reacted to a car stopping near her residence. Under normal circumstances, this mundane event would not have been deemed to have been suspicious, but in the light of the gasser scare, it took on a new, potentially sinister meaning [41]. The *Roanake Times* captured the increasing mood of frustration and skepticism:

> Residents at 316 Howbert avenue, Wasena, detected strange fumes near a furnace register about 8:25 but no one suffered any ill effects and police said they believed the fumes had come from the furnace. No one was seen or heard about the house before the odor was detected...
>
> Three reports were received between 10 and 11 o'clock...at 551 Washington avenue, S.W.--both occupants and police detected fumes, but they came from a thawing automobile radiator which contained alcohol. Several persons were playing bridge when the fumes were noticed. Police found that an automobile had been driven into a garage at the rear of the house and the smell of alcohol was decidedly noticeable.
>
> A resident at 311 Broadway, South Roanoke, entered a bedroom and detected a peculiar odor. Police said they failed to find any trace of a noxious gas.
>
> Residents at 811 and 813 Shenandoah avenue, N.W., noted a peculiar odor about 11 o'clock. Police said they believed that the occupants had smelled sulphur in coal smoke from passing trains. [41]

Amid a flurry of false alarms, reports of gas attacks stopped in both Virginia counties after the night of February 11, 1934. An editorial appeared in the *Roanoke Times* on February 14 entitled "Roanoke has no gasser." It indicated that the paper had been suspicious of the gasser right from the start "but it seemed best to permit the police to go ahead and investigate without whatever handicap they might be under were cold water to be thrown on their search in advance." Whether or not this was true, many of the earlier reports in the paper, presented the existence of the gasser as a reality. This often included dramatic headlines. There can be no question that the paper played a major role in fueling the outbreak, but conversely, once it began to report on the growing skepticism of authorities, this helped to create a wave of counter-suggestibility and bring an end to the case.

The Mad Gasser of Mattoon, Illinois

One of the most famous episodes of mass psychogenic illness in the twentieth century occurred in Mattoon, Illinois, during September 1944, about 10 ½ years after the Virginia outbreak. It has become a staple in introductory textbooks on psychology and sociology as a classic example of mass hysteria. The fear of gas attacks increased with the onset of World War II and played a pivotal role in the outbreak. Although at the time of the Mattoon incident neither side had used chemical weapons for fear of retaliation both the Allied and Axis governments had stockpiled chemical weapons and soldiers and civilians were constantly warned about the possibility of a gas attack. Articles regularly appeared in the mass media on chemical warfare. Rumors of the Japanese use of chemical weapons prompted calls for retaliation in the American press. As the tide of war in Europe began to turn in favor of the Allies in 1944, there was great concern that an increasingly desperate Germany might turn to gas warfare [42]. Magazines of this period were filled with chilling stories about the 'poison gas peril' [43–45]. It was feared that in the face of the June

6, 1944 D-Day invasion of Normandy, desperate German commanders might unleash poison gas attacks on civilian targets in the American mainland [46]. It may be no coincidence then, that the 'mad gasser' appeared within 2 1/2 months of D-Day.

Mattoon was a typical Midwestern American city with about 17,000 inhabitants in 1944. It is located in central Illinois and surrounded by farmland. On a typical tree-lined street in the north of the city on September 1, 1944, Aline Kearney had just gone to bed with her 3-year-old daughter, Dorothy Ellen. Her sister Martha who was staying at the house while her husband was serving in the Navy was in bed in the front room, and Mrs. Kearney's other daughter and her sister's son were sleeping in the back room. While reading in bed Mrs. Kearney noticed a "sickening sweet odor" that she initially thought was coming from a bed of flowers just below her window. She called Martha to see if she could smell the odor, but Martha reported that she didn't smell anything. As the odor became more prominent, Mrs. Kerney felt "paralyzed" in her legs and lower body and she noted a tightness and dryness in her throat. She called out for her sister and when Martha came she also noticed the smell. She called the neighbors who phoned the police but when they arrived, they found nothing. Meanwhile, when her husband Burt, a taxi driver, returned home he thought he saw a man near the bedroom window but when he took chase, he melted into the night. He was tall with dark clothes and a tight-fitting cap. Mrs. Kerney's paralysis resolved within half an hour, while her daughter who also taken ill, had both recovered by the next morning. Police hypothesized that someone had sprayed the bedroom with an anesthetic, possibly ether or chloroform. The only large circulation newspaper in Mattoon, the *Daily Journal-Gazette* published a sensational article the next evening with the headline: "Anesthetic Prowler on Loose." They described how Mrs. Kearney and her daughter were the victims of a gas attack and attempted robbery but the prowler failed to get into the house. After reading the story other Mattoon families began reporting similar attacks on their homes – some even happening *before* the Kearney attack [47–51].

Mr. and Mrs. Orban Raef reported to the police that they had been asleep in their bedroom the night before the attack on the Kearney residence when at about 3 a.m. they smelled something strange coming from the bedroom window. They each developed "the same feeling of paralysis" and were ill for about an hour and a half. Mrs. Olive Brown claimed that she and her daughter had been attacked by the gasser a few months earlier and had similar symptoms to the others but she did not report the episode since it seemed so farfetched. Mrs. George Rider reported that the gasser had attacked her house on the same night as the Kearney incident. Mrs. Rider told authorities that she had drunk "several pots" of coffee while waiting for her husband to return home from work. She then went to lay in bed with her two small children when she heard a noise like a "plop," followed shortly by a strange smell that made her feel dizzy like she was floating. The bedroom window was closed because the 2-year-old had a cold. With the dizziness, she developed numbness and tingling of the hands and legs. On the same night, a few blocks from the Rider house a woman reported that the gasser had forced fumes with a sickeningly sweet smell through a bedroom window causing her children to vomit [52].

The next attack occurred 4 days after the Kearney attack and was even more bizarre than the previously reported incidents. Mrs. Beulah Cordes found an approximately 6 by 9-inch cloth lying on her front porch and noticing a wet spot in the center of it, she picked it up and took a whiff. She staggered and screamed, later reporting that it felt like an electric shock went through her legs into her toes. "It was a feeling of paralysis." Her husband helped her inside where she had difficulty swallowing or speaking and remained sick for the next 2 hours. She later speculated that even though she didn't hear anything, the gasser was probably trying to anesthetize her dog when he was frightened away. The cloth was sent to the Police Crime Laboratory in Springfield where a chemical analysis showed no trace of any gas so it was assumed that it must have evaporated. When contacted by the press, U. S. Army chemical warfare experts suggested that the mystery gas might have been chloropicrin, poisonous gas with a sweet odor that is often used to exterminate rodents [53]. The mayor of Mattoon, who also happened to be a doctor, suggested the possibility oil of mustard, which has a pungent smell and could cause a burning and tingling sensation if placed on the skin, while experts from the Chemical Warfare Service in Chicago favored chloropicrin [54]. But how would it be sprayed through windows without leaving a trace?

By September 6, the number of gassing reports was overwhelming Mattoon's modest police force consisting of two officers and eight patrolmen, so the Commissioner of Public Safety sent an urgent message for help to the State Department of Safety. Just as with the Virginia incident, vigilante gangs of men and boys patrolled the city streets with clubs and guns on foot and in cars and trucks [55]. One woman, whose husband was on duty in the Army, loaded his shotgun for protection and accidentally blew a hole through the kitchen wall [56]. As a police car shot off into the night to answer a presumed gasser attack, it was followed by a procession of civilian vehicles anxious to see a gasser victim. Police were understandably concerned about the possibility innocent people being injured or killed, so the chief ordered officers to arrest chasers [55].

On the weekend of September 9 and 10, dozens of gas attacks were reported throughout the city, stretching police thin. Nights were terrifying as residents grouped together in selected homes and the men stood guard in shifts throughout the night. Perhaps the most dramatic and vivid claim involved two sisters – Frances and Maxine Smith who reported a series of attacks in their home. In their September 9 edition, the *Gazette* reported the claims as fact. "The first infiltration of gas caught them in their beds. Gasping and choking, they awoke and soon felt partial paralysis grip their legs and arms. Later, while awake, the other attacks came and they saw a thin, blue smoke-like vapor spreading throughout the room. …Just before the gas with its 'flower-like' odor came pouring into the room they heard a strange 'buzzing' sound outside the house and expressed the belief that the sound probably was made by the 'madman's spraying apparatus' in operation" [53]. During the weekend, two more women were rushed to hospital after apparent gassings, only to be diagnosed with "nervous tension" [57]. Most victims reported that the odor was sweet, even flower-like but others said it resembled the smell of ether or gasoline.

In some cases, a noise alone could trigger symptoms. The symptoms were remarkably variable including abdominal pain, nausea, vomiting, dryness of the mouth and throat, smothering and choking, numbness and tingling, and weakness and paralysis. In most instances, the symptoms lasted from a few hours to a day and only a few were hospitalized. Physicians who examined the patients could not find any objective abnormalities on physical examination or laboratory tests; some noted the presence of anxiety and nervous tension. A front-page article in the *Chicago Herald-American* on September 10 entitled "MATTOON GETS JITTERS FROM GAS ATTACKS" reflected the reporter's vivid imagination more than the actual facts but no doubt increased the general fear and anxiety. "Groggy as Londoners under protracted aerial blitzing, this town's bewildered citizens reeled today under the repeated attacks of a mad anesthetist who has sprayed a deadly nerve gas into 13 homes and has knocked out 27 known victims. Seventy others dashing to the area in response to the alarm, fell under the influence of the gas last night. All skepticism has vanished and Mattoon grimly concedes it must fight haphazardly against a demented phantom adversary who has been seen only fleetingly and so far has evaded traps laid by the city and state police and posses of townsmen" [58]. The next day the same newspaper ran a headline with one and a half inch bold letters: **STATE HUNTS GAS MADMAN.**

Everyone had a pet theory on who the mad gasser might be. Initially, many thought it was a prankster but as the number and severity of attacks increased, the possibility of a demented high school chemistry student was entertained. Others thought it was a mad scientist experimenting with a new gas developed in his secret laboratory. Many thought it must have something to do with chemical warfare: an escaped Nazi or Japanese prisoner or possibly a disgruntled ex-soldier trained in chemical weapons. Witnesses could not agree on whether the gasser was tall and thin or short and fat. Most thought it was a man but one lady was convinced that the gasser was a woman. A 55-year-old widow, Bertha Bence was sleeping in the front room of her cottage when she heard a strange "whirring noise" coming through a partly open window. She felt nauseated and lightheaded like she might faint. After crying out, her three sons immediately ran outside after the gasser. The oldest, Orville, thought he saw someone disappearing into an alley. The next morning they found high-heel shoe prints outside the bedroom window and concluded that the gasser was a woman dressed as a man [59]. Just as with the finding of high-heel shoe prints in the Virginia case, the idea of a woman with high-heel shoes dashing about in the night seemed far-fetched. Undoubtedly, the most bizarre story of all was the ape-man sighting reported by Mrs. Edna James, a fortune teller, and owner of a men's hotel. Mrs. James claimed that she smelled a strange odor and went to investigate only to encounter an ape-like man with long arms reaching out, holding a spray gun. He doused her with three clouds of gas causing her arms and legs to go numb. She claimed she saw the ape-man a second time 2 days later in the lobby of her hotel but several other guests who were present reported seeing nothing [60].

After that chaotic weekend, Mattoon was flooded with law enforcement officers determined to catch the gasser. The chief of the Illinois State Police sent five squad cars, each with two armed officers and a volunteer to provide local knowledge.

Nearby Urbana sent three police officers to patrol the streets at night. The FBI sent two agents who focused on identifying the type of gas that the "madman" used [61, 62]. Police were suspicious that several of the reports over the weekend were false alarms and on Monday a frantic woman called them to report that she had been gassed in broad daylight. As the officers converged on the house they discovered that she had accidentally spilled a bottle of nail polish remover. The Mattoon police chief, C. Eugene Cole had seen enough. He announced that the whole idea of a mad anesthetist was a mistake from the beginning. It was a case of mass hysteria. He speculated that the odors were probably coming from the Atlas Imperial Diesel Engine Company that produced army shell casings as shifting winds carried them wafting throughout the city. Atlas officials rebuked that idea, pointing out that none of their employees noticed fumes or became sick. Cole then suggested that the odors could have come from other Mattoon factories using chemicals.

The majority of Mattoon's citizens initially rejected the notion of mass hysteria, suggesting instead that the police were trying to cover up their incompetence. A few days earlier, when Chief Cole initially hinted that some of the gas attacks may have been triggered by "nerves," the Mattoon *Journal-Gazette* responded with a scathing editorial critical of the Chief and anyone who did not take the attacks seriously: "One of the principal difficulties throughout has been that the whole matter was taken lightly. It was easy to say, 'Oh, its just imagination!' and shrug the whole thing off with a disdainful air" [63]. The Illinois State Attorney, William K. Kidwell, considered Cole's hysteria hypothesis "ridiculous" and suggested that the police had let the situation get out of control [64]. Meanwhile, the investigation proceeded and word leaked that police were narrowing in on a wealthy eccentric with a laboratory in his basement living in the area near where many of the attacks had occurred. He had been a brilliant student in high school and college but recently had become a recluse and neighbors thought he was demented. The notion that a mad scientist was threatening the community was popular but there was no evidence tying the man to the attacks. At the same time, State Police were busy calling mental hospitals to see if any recently released patient had an obsession with poison gas [65]. In an attempt to identify the substance used in the attacks, everyone involved in a gas attack was asked to smell tiny amounts of various chemicals including tear gas, mustard gas, chloropicrin, methol chloride, and Lewisite to see which chemical was closest to the one used by the gasser. Chloropicrin won the contest but was by no means a unanimous choice. Of course, in retrospect, there really weren't any poisonous gasses that could account for the symptoms, their course and the lack of objective findings. Even a slight exposure to a gas such as chloropicrin would cause breathing difficulties and eye irritation that would be obvious and require medical attention. The examining physicians should have seen something. Further, most gases would linger and should have been readily detected by authorities.

And then the reports of gas attacks abruptly stopped. This occurred as police pushed the mass hysteria explanation and the press began to join the act. The *Decatur Herald* made fun of their neighbor Mattoonites noting: "At this season of the year odors are sniffed not only by individuals but by entire communities. Our neighbors in Mattoon sniffed their town into newspaper headlines from coast to coast" [66]. The Mattoon *Journal-Gazette* which obviously played a major role in starting and propagating the whole incident decided to join in the fun suggesting in an editorial that "Decatur's famous odors, carried Mattoonward by the wind" was the cause of the gas mania. Although they admitted that mass hysteria took over as public fear spiralled out of control, they still insisted that the early cases were the victim of a gasser who was not apprehended because of police incompetence [66]. On September 22, 1944, the *Chicago Herald American*, another newspaper that had stoked the flames of the Mattoon gas mania, published an interview with psychiatrist Dr. Harold Hulbert, who had studied the Mattoon incident. He compared the Mattoon episode to that of the Salem witch trials of 1692 and suggested that "the same forces which created the recent terror (in Mattoon) have at one time or another manifested themselves in nearly every American community, sometimes with tragic, sometimes with comic results" [67].

After a brief flurry of publicity in the fall of 1944, the Mattoon gasser episode was largely forgotten in the wake of the rapidly moving events involving the war in Europe and the Far East. Interest in the gasser panic was rekindled in 1945 when an undergraduate student at the University of Illinois, Donald Johnson, published an article describing the event in the *Journal of Abnormal and Social Psychology*. Johnson outlined the gas attacks in detail, tabulating the numbers involved in the many different circumstances. Remarkably, Johnson concluded that nearly all the victims of the gas attacks were women, presumably because he was taught that only women were prone to hysteria. It was true that many of the men from the community were off fighting in the war so many households were predominantly female, but in several of the attacks where husbands and wives were together, both suffered the same symptoms but only the wives were counted as victims by Johnson. Furthermore, several male journalists from Chicago and other nearby cities reported developing lingering symptoms after visiting the site of an attack but were not reported as victims.

Voodoo Assailants

Many contemporary phantom attacker cases involve the supposed use of supernatural powers. Such cases are common across part of Africa, Asia, and the Caribbean. In Malaysia, outbreaks of psychogenic illness are arguably the most common of any place on earth [68–71]. Cases are often attributed to attacks by a host of creatures from popular Malay culture including the *jinn* (creatures mentioned in the Koran), fairy-like *toyl* beings, and *hantus*, ghosts from Malay folklore [72–74]. The belief is so widespread and strong that many people offer their services in the Yellow pages, newspaper classified ads, and online, claiming to be able to remove spells, and make love charms, or to place curses on people. Outbreaks of motor hysteria in repressive school settings that manifest as demonic possession are very common across the African continent. We have collected several hundred cases from media reports during the twenty-first century alone.

A rare Western example of this type occurred in April 1976 when 15 girls at the Sand Flat School in Mount Pleasant, Mississippi, began to act strangely and collapsed. The students would roll around, "writhing and kicking before passing out" [75]. Some were screaming, "Don't let it get me!" or "Get it off!" then passing out. Police initially suspected that the girls had been taking drugs, but tests ruled this out. Many parents blamed voodoo. It was eventually diagnosed as a case of 'mass hysteria' triggered by the local belief in supernatural powers after a group of girls believed they had been hexed by a rival classmate in an attempt to win the affection of a boy. The girls grew anxious and when they began to exhibit trance-like states, the fear of "black magic" swept quickly through the rest of the group, only serving to confirm the reality of the 'attack.' The belief in voodoo magic was so great within the community that before the week was out, nearly 300 of the school's 900 students were absent from school fearing that they too could become the next victims [76, 77]. One of the affected girls, 14-year-old Shirley Benton said, "My head was hurting bad. It wasn't like a headache. It felt like something was sticking in it. …I couldn't get enough air. Then I fell out – fainted." This description appears to be an indirect reference to the use of voodoo dolls. Authorities later learned that some of the girls had a previous history of fainting spells, which was believed to have prompted the spread of symptoms [78].

Phantom Slashers and Monsters

Many episodes involving imaginary assailants in Western countries are lacking in somatic complaints and are driven by cultural traditions and media reports in conjunction with human perceptual fallibility, which is highly unreliable and conditioned by a person's mental outlook. As a result, in ambiguous, stressful situations "inference can perform the work of perception by filling in missing information in instances where perception is either inefficient or inadequate" [79]. A famous example of an imaginary assailant began in May 1956, when fear swept through the island nation of Taiwan after media reports that a crazed slasher was on the loose, randomly cutting people with a razor blade. Sociologist Norman Jacobs was teaching in the capital city of Taipei at the time and studied the episode by examining the press coverage. The two major hotspots of the scare were Taipei, and the city of Keelung 40 miles to the north, where residents feared that they or their children would be the slasher's next victim. News of the maniac's existence first appeared in the press on May 4, when it was reported that several children, ranging in age from 6 months to 8 years, had been attacked by a razor-wielding fiend. It was claimed that the attacks had been occurring for up to 3 months, with one paper, the *China Post*, stating that there had been as many as 30 victims. There did not appear to be any pattern to the incidents, with people supposedly having been slashed on the back, arms, and head. Two papers – the *China Post* and the *Hong Kong Standard*, reported that one of the victims had been castrated and killed [80, p 319]. The matter had been brought to the attention of the press on May 3 after police decided to open a formal investigation upon hearing rumors of attacks and because of an incident that had occurred that morning, involving a woman carrying a knife. The woman was found wandering in the city center and held for questioning as she hailed from an aboriginal Taiwanese tribe that was once known for head-hunting. She had apparently had an argument with a pedicab driver and was brandishing the knife for protection after she claimed he had threatened her [80]. Many possible motives were discussed, including the theory that the attacks were the result of a blood ritual, reflecting a local belief that drawing blood from a child is good luck. Other opinions ranged from the possibility that there was a sexual sadist on the loose, to the slashings being a smokescreen cover to divert attention from jewelry thieves [80, p 320].

Amid the flurry of press reports, one oddly stood out: no one had actually observed the slasher in the act. Residents could not even agree on whether the culprit was a male or female. While the rumors appear to have given rise to sensational press coverage, the subsequent press reports and their ambiguous nature, appear to have spawned even more rumors. Before long, it was evident that people going about their everyday life, began to redefine a variety of ordinary events and circumstances, within an extraordinary framework – that of the slasher. On May 4 two children were reportedly slashed, although the circumstances were vague. In one instance, an 11-year-old boy noticed a cut on his arm but could not recall how it happened. The other incident involved a 2-year-old boy who suffered a laceration to his leg while playing near his house. The Police Chief held a press conference and criticized the press for inaccurately reporting that a slasher victim had died. However, he added to anxieties when he refused to deny that deaths had occurred. At this point, police were engaged in an all-out effort to solve the mystery by situating several plain-clothes detectives in market areas, schools, theatres, and other public places [80, p 321].

On May 5, authorities said that they had been unable to confirm a single slashing. The next day, one of the cases investigated by the police involved a child who claimed to have been slashed 3 days earlier in her father's shop. Authorities went to the shop, examined the scene and determined that she had actually suffered a bruised ankle while playing with an iron rod. Three new claims came from Keelung, where there were three separate incidents involving youngsters who, while on their way home from school, claimed to have been slashed. To underscore the tension over the scare, the country's chief prosecutor ordered police and court officials across the nation to thoroughly investigate any alleged attacks in their area [80, p 323]. On May 7 police noticed a crowd reading a note on a fence. The note had drawings of knives, a signature and a local address in Keelung. Police then noticed a boy acting suspiciously. They matched his handwriting to the note and he confessed that he had gotten into an argument with an acquaintance while playing cards, and was trying to get him in trouble [80, p 324].

The scare peaked on May 11 when there was a sensational development. Police appeared to have caught the slasher after arresting a "woman in red" in the northwest sector of Taipei after she was reported to have taken a razor blade and slashed a 9-month-old baby while being held in her mother's arms. The mother said she was on the street when suddenly her baby cried after being struck by an object from behind. She noticed the baby was bleeding. Looking around, she saw a girl in a red jacket and cried out. The girl fled, the mother in pursuit. Bystanders joined in. The girl dropped her red coat on the road, threw away a small package and tried to lose herself in the crowd. Police arrested the girl and took her in for questioning. It seemed that at long last, they had captured the slasher. As they began to ask her questions, a mob formed outside the station. The woman said that as it was about to rain, she began to open her umbrella and it accidentally caught on the baby's sleeve. When the mother cried out, she panicked and took off. The woman said she was petrified because she had been carrying a razor which she used in her job as a seamstress, but she feared that she could be mistaken for the slasher. The mother contradicted the woman's story, claiming that she had the umbrella in one hand and the razor in the other. She then reminded police that the razor in the package was discovered wrapped in paper and thus could not have been used as a weapon. The only 'weapons' that she possessed were long fingernails and an umbrella. When a doctor was called in to examine the baby's wound, he determined that a razor could not have produced it and that the umbrella scenario seemed plausible. The mob was dispersed and the girl was released [80, p 325].

On May 12, police made a dramatic announcement: they had solved the slasher case. Based on their investigation of 21 cases, they concluded that the episode was a result of hoaxing and mass suggestion. Of the 21 claims reported to police, "five were innocent false reports, seven were self-inflicted cuts, eight were due to cuts other than razors, and one was a complete fantasy." It was evident that the 'slashings' were the result of inadvertent contact in public places – the type of contact that occurs every day and under ordinary circumstances would have garnered little notice. For example, one man told a doctor in minute detail how he had been slashed by a man in his 30s with a mysterious black bag. Upon examining the wound, the doctor determined that the wound could not have been caused by a razor, and the likely culprit had been a dull object. The man then admitted that he could not recall how he got the cut, but assumed that it may have been slasher-related due to "all the talk going around about razor slashings" [80, p 322]. In another instance, a physician inadvertently created a victim when an elderly man sought medical treatment for a lacerated wrist. The doctor contacted police and the man noted that he first noticed the blood at the same time he had been touched by a stranger. The police examined the 'slash' and concluded that it was an old injury that had likely reopened after the man had innocently scratched it [80, p 322]. In another case, this one involving a falsified report, a 17-year-old boy had accidentally cut his elbow on a piece of broken glass. But instead of being admonished for carelessness by his mother, he claimed to have been slashed. The false report was uncovered after someone who had witnessed the boy cut himself, read about the slashings in the press. In another case, a neighbor had reported that a boy had been slashed while playing nearby. While the mother embellished the story, a closer investigation revealed beyond any doubt, that the boy had accidentally cut himself on a waste can [80, p 322].

The Montreal 'Slasher'

A remarkably similar episode took place in 1954, when police in Montreal, Canada, determined that most if not all of the victims of a crazed slasher targeting women's legs during late January, were the likely result of "mass hysteria." The 'attacks' typically took place at stops for streetcars or buses during rush hour, near the city center. On January 29, the *New York Times* reported that according to Canadian police, the 'phantom slasher,' appeared to have been "largely a case of mass hysteria. Police said that many of the attacks were false and that some of the wounds were self-inflicted" [81]. The next day the *Chicago Tribune* reported that "Police and psychologists asked Montreal newspapers and radio stations… to help combat 'mass hysteria' which has seized women and children who fear the attacks of a phantom slasher in this city…" Meanwhile, police noted that they had determined that at least four of the complaints were "fake." A fifth incident turned out to be a case of mistaken identity when a police detective tried to arrest a suspect loitering on a street corner – it was another detective [82]. No one was ever convicted of the attacks, which soon subsided and were largely forgotten about.

Monkey Man 'Attacks' in India

A classic non-Western example of a phantom assailant took place in New Delhi, India during May 2001. The episode highlights the importance of cultural and religious beliefs. Many residents in the eastern part of the city were living in fear of a creature that was said to have been part man, part monkey. Dubbed the 'monkey man,' the creature was reported to have long claws and supernatural qualities such as super strength, and the ability to leap great distances. It would attack its prey almost exclusively at night, with most incidents focused in East Delhi after sunset while people slept outside to escape the oppressive heat due to a series of ongoing power blackouts [83]. A journalist for *Time Asia*, Michael Fathers, captured the atmosphere of escalating fear: "Wandering bands of vigilantes guard neighborhoods with wooden cudgels, daggers, field-hockey sticks, ceremonial swords and pikes made from butchers' cleavers. In the early hours, police fire flares over cultivated ground to see if the Monkey Man is hiding in the darkness. The area's 500-strong police force has been tripled. Some legislators are demanding the central government send in elite commandos to deal with what they call 'the crisis.' A bounty of $1,100 has been put on his head" [84].

At least two people died in incidents that police attributed to the scare. In one case, a pregnant women fell down a stairway in the dark trying to flee the creature after neighbors shouted that the monkey man was nearby [85]. In another incident, a man was awakened by the sounds of screeching, assumed he was about to be attacked by the monkey man, and in his haste to get away, inadvertently leaped off a one-story building [86]. One witness described their encounter in broken English:

"I open the curtain and I saw a hand." Few people claimed to get a clear view of the mysterious creature. A description by another witness was typically vague: "Then I heard a noise, a noise like a monkey makes, and I started running towards the stairs and he chased me. Then I tripped over something in the hall and fell down the stairs. He didn't follow, but I could see he had a dark face and an iron hand" [87]. The ambiguous nature of the 'encounters' was highlighted by the variation in descriptions by eyewitnesses: anywhere from 3 to 6 feet in tall, although some said it was as small as a cat!

The existence of such a creature would seem ridiculous to most people growing up in Western countries, but not so in India. The outbreak coincided with the airing of *Hanuman*, a TV series about a Hindu monkey god that just so happened to possess superhuman strength and an incredible leaping ability [84]. Earlier in the year concerns were expressed over the exploding population of monkeys in the city, creating havoc [88]. Monkeys were common in the area of the sightings and attacks, while many local residents who were forced to sleep on their balconies and rooftops at night to escape the heatwave amid power cuts, likely felt vulnerable. Within this environment of fear and uncertainty, peoples' imaginations ran wild as they began to misperceive mundane occurrences such as monkeys or shadows, which became redefined as an attack. One victim told authorities: "The creature had its hands on my thighs when I woke up. It looked like a langur [a type of monkey]...When Rehena, my mother, picked up a broomstick, it jumped out of the balcony" [89]. Many people were beaten up by mobs after being mistaken for the attackers. In one case, a four-foot tall Indian mystic was cornered, beaten and taken to the local police station where it was established that he was innocent [85].

The events of May 16 were typical, with police receiving about 40 calls reporting attacks or sightings of the elusive creature. When they arrived on the scene of one 'assault,' it was clear that the victim had been bitten by a rat [90]. Several 'fresh wounds' attributed to the Monkey Man were later determined to have been old wounds that had been reopened in an effort to gain attention [91]. After 3 weeks of investigating vague, shadowy sightings, looking at ambiguous scratch marks, and uncovering a number of hoaxes, a police investigation concluded that there was no monkey man [92]. A study of the episode was conducted by local doctors and published in the *Indian Journal of Medical Sciences*. They found that the scope of the scare was remarkable. Between May 10 and 25, 397 phone calls were made to police in Delhi to report an attack by a monkey-like creature. They also examined the records of 51 patients presenting at their teaching hospital in Delhi, with 'attack' wounds. They found that where the time of the attack was given, all but one was under the cover of darkness, while 94 percent of patients were poorly educated. Most attacks happened after power outages, and most of the victims had been asleep at the time of the incident and the electricity was not working, hence, there was poor lighting. This is consistent with injuries that were deemed to have been from accidental falls and other injuries in the dark. Supporting this assessment were the descriptions. The study found that of the cases examined, not one of the victims got a clear look at their attacker [93].

'Attack' at Frog Hollow

Some cases involving imaginary assailants have turned out to be remarkable in terms of the extent to which entire communities can fool themselves, especially in situations involving ambiguity and fear. A classic example of this took place during the American French and Indian War of 1754–1763. During this period, occasional enemy raiding parties across the British colonies resulted in jittery colonists. It was within this context that soon after midnight in July 1758, the inhabitants of Windham, Connecticut, were awakened by mysterious noises. The menfolk loaded their muskets and prepared to fend off what was believed to be an imminent attack by a French and Indian raiding party. The tension soon built to unbearable levels the strange sounds grew louder. Many in the group could distinctly hear the Indian screeches and war-whoops as they prepared for the attack. A local newspaper of the period, known as a broadsheet, reported that "At intervals, many supposed they could distinguish the calling out of the particular names, as of Cols. Dyer and Elderkin two eminent lawyers, and this increased the general terror." With the strange sounds echoing through the air, soon residents rushed "from every house, the tumult in the air still increasing – old and young, male and female, poured forth into the streets" [94]. The next morning a scouting party was sent out to check on the position of the Indians and soon discovered the source: with the community in the midst of a drought, bullfrogs had been fighting over the last remaining small patch of water puddles of what was left of a pond. Many of the frogs were dead [95]. The extraordinary nature of the sounds during the incident may owe to atmospheric conditions (warm and foggy), and the geography. Frog Pond is located only 1 mile from the Village of Windham, separated by a sloping hill. For whatever reason related to either the weather or internal biology, they were particularly loud on that fateful summer's early morning. The incident has been embraced by the town having a frog on their official seal and has been the subject of poems, postcards, songs, and even an opera.

References

1. Dorsey C. My heavenly heart. New York: Kensington; 1995. p. 51.
2. Stone JR. The Routledge book of proverbs. New York: Routledge; 2006.
3. Bullard TE. Mysteries in the eye of the beholder: ufos and their correlates as a folkloric theme past and present [dissertation]. Bloomington: Indiana University; 1982. p. 10–1.
4. Nickell J. Real-life x-files. Lexington: University of Kentucky Press; 2001. p. 12.
5. Bartholomew RE. Redefining epidemic hysteria: an example from Sweden. Acta Psychiatr Scand. 1993;88:178–82.
6. Bartholomew RE, Dawes G, Liljegren A, Svahn C. The Swedish ghost rocket delusion of 1946: anatomy of a moral panic. Fortean Studies (London). 1999;6:64–74.
7. Durbin K. Handling of school emergency examined. Columbian (Vancouver, WA). 2001;Sect C:1.
8. Martin MG. Palawan school cancelled after 15 students 'possessed by evil spirits.' Philippines Lifestyle News. 24 Feb 2018.
9. Satanism scare see school shut down. The Chronicle (Bulawayo, Zimbabwe). 27 Mar 2018.

10. Pupils rushed to church after mass hysteria closes two Cebu schools. Philippines Lifestyle News. 22 Jun 2018.
11. Martin MG. cebu schoolgirls fall victim to demonic possession after seeing ghosts. Philippines Lifestyle News. 13 Jul 2018.
12. Martin MG. Priests rush to Siquijor Island after schoolchildren 'possessed by demons.' Philippines Lifestyle News. 17 Oct 2018.
13. Ambrad L. 14 students in Dalaguete 'possessed' by spirits. The Freeman (Cebu, Philippines). 11 Jul 2018.
14. Sotto J. 13 students 'possessed' by evil spirit in Danao City. Cebu Daily News. 13 Jul 2018.
15. Antojado L. Evil spirits 'possess' 46 students in Ronda, Argao. The Freeman (Manila). 24 Jun 2018.
16. School closed after satanism scare. The Zimbabwe Mail (Harare). 25 Feb 2018.
17. 'Black figure' 'haunts' catholic school. Bulawayo 24 News (Bulawayo, Zimbabwe). 16 Mar 2018.
18. Kolyangha M. Parents dump 45 pupils at Budaka police station over suspected demon attacks. Daily Monitor (Kampala, Uganda). 9 Oct 2018.
19. Nabukenya J. Mityana school resumes classes after suspected demons cast out. The Daily Monitor (Kampala, Uganda). October 22 2018.
20. Okertchiri J. Nungua SHS students collapse under strange circumstances. Daily Guide (Accra, Ghana). 4 Jul 2018.
21. Alias NA. Kelantan school hit by mass hysteria for 3rd time. New Straits Times (Kuala Lumpur, Malaysia). 23 Jul 2018.
22. Mass Hysteria grips girls in Jalpaiguri school, parents consult shaman instead of doctor. Newsmen (Bengal, India). 19 Sept 2018.
23. Rahman K. Nearly 30 children suffer 'hysteria' after playing with a ouija board at a boarding school in Peru. The Daily Mail (London). 26 Sept 2018.
24. Bartholomew RE. Little green men, meowing nuns and head-hunting panics. Jefferson: McFarland; 2001. p. 81–94.
25. Bartholomew RE, Victor J. A social psychological theory of collective anxiety attacks. Sociol Q. 2004;45(2):229–48.
26. Ladendorf R, Bartholomew RE. The mad gasser of Mattoon: how the press created an imaginary chemical weapons attack. Skept Inq. 2002;26(4):50–3, 58.
27. Gas 'attack' on family is probed. fumes at night fell girl and make others ill at Haymakertown home... Roanoke Times (Roanoke, VA). 24 Dec 1933. p. 13.
28. Gas attacks...second reported from Cloverdale. Roanoke Times. 27 Dec 1933. p. 2.
29. Stealthy gasser is active again. Troutville man is latest victim... Roanoke Times. 29 Dec 1933. p. 2.
30. ...Finds woman's track. Roanoke Times. 29 Dec 1933. p. 2.
31. ...Reports chlorine used. Roanoke Times. 21 Jan 1934. p. 15.
32. Continue search for 'gas' clues. Officers' test eliminates chlorine–inhabitants are highly keyed. Roanoke Times. 31 Jan 1934. p. 2.
33. Gas throwers make new foray...reward of $500 authorized... Roanoke Times. 30 Jan 1934. p. 2.
34. ...Hoax angle taken up. Roanoke Times. 30 Jan 1934.
35. ...Fears injury to innocent. Roanoke Times. 31 Jan 1934. p. 2.
36. ...Sheriff 'from Missouri.' Roanoke Times. 6 Feb 1934. p. 2.
37. Mysterious gas thrower visits home at Vinton. Roanoke Times. 6 Feb 1934. p. 3.
38. 2 new 'gassings' puzzle to police. Lynchburg News (Lynchburg, VA). 7 Feb 1934. p. 3.
39. Rorer Avenue Home Target of Mysterious Gas Attack... Roanoke Times. 8 Feb 1934. pp. 1, 4.
40. ...Gas not identified. Roanoke Times. 8 Feb 1934. p. 4.
41. 5 attacks by mystery gasser keep police busy. reports of nocturnal visits come from widely separated spots. Roanoke Times. 9 Feb 1934. pp. 1, 4.
42. Marshall J. We are ready with gas if the Axis turns on the gas. Collier's. 1943;112:21.
43. Lindley EK. Thoughts on the use of gas in warfare. Newsweek. 1943;22:24.
44. Sanders V. Our army's defense against poison gas. Pop Sci. 1945;146:106–11.

45. Scott EW. Role of the public health laboratory in gas defense. Am J Public Health. 1944;275-8(March):34.
46. Brown F. Chemical warfare: a study in restraints. Princeton: Princeton University Press; 1968. p. 244.
47. Anesthetic prowler on loose. The Daily Journal-Gazette. 2 Sept 1944. p. 1.
48. Show how they were gassed. Chicago Herald-American. 10 Sept 1944. p. 10.
49. Alley E. Illness of first gas 'victim' blamed for wave of hysteria in Mattoon. Chicago Herald-American. 17 Sept 1944. p. 3.
50. Chicago psychiatrist analyzes Mattoon gas hysteria. Chicago Herald-American. 17 Sept 1944. p. 3.
51. Johnson DM. The 'phantom anesthetist' of Mattoon: a field study of mass hysteria. J Abnorm Psychol. 1945;40:175–86.
52. Mattoon's phantom 'suggestive' fear. Chicago Herald-American. 21 Sept 1944. p. 2.
53. 'Mad gasser' adds six victims! 5 women and boy latest overcome. The Daily Journal-Gazette. 9 Sept 1944. p. 1.
54. Safety agent to aid police in 'gas' case. The Daily Journal-Gazette. 6 Sept 1944. p. 6.
55. To all citizens of Mattoon. The Daily Journal-Gazette. 11 Sept 1944. p. 1.
56. Sidelights of 'mad gasser's' strange case. The Daily Journal-Gazette. 12 Sept 1944. p. 4.
57. ...Two Women Believed Victims Examined at Hospital. The Daily Journal-Gazette. 11 Sept 1944. p. 1.
58. Mattoon gets jitters from gas attacks. Chicago Herald-American. 10 Sept 1944. p. 1.
59. Suspect woman gas terrorist. find prints of high-heeled shoes. Chicago Herald-American. 15 Sept 1944. p. 3.
60. M'Hugh L. Ape man clue at Mattoon. Chicago Herald-American. 16 Sept 1944. p. 3.
61. Ballenger C. FBI at Mattoon as gas prowler attacks 5 more. Chicago Daily Tribune. 10 Sept 1944. p. 15.
62. Many prowler reports; few real. city calmer after wild week-end. Daily Journal-Gazette. 11 Sept 1944. p. 1.
63. Mattoon's mad anesthetist. Daily Journal-Gazette. 8 Sept 1944. p. 2.
64. Ballenger C. Assail police for calling gas scare a hoax. The Chicago Daily Tribune. 14 Sept 1944. p. 18.
65. Press search for Mattoon prowler. Illinois State Journal (Springfield, IL). 12 Sept 1944. p. 5.
66. The 'perfumed city' speaks.' The Daily Journal-Gazette. 20 Sept 1944. p. 2.
67. Alley E. Mattoon terror like Salem witch-hunt. Chicago Herald-American. 22 Sept 1944. p. 4.
68. Tan E. Epidemic hysteria. Med J Malaya. 1963;18(2):72–6.
69. Teoh J, Soewondo S, Sidharta M. Epidemic hysteria in Malaysia: an illustrative episode. Psychiatry. 1975;8(3):258–68.
70. Lee RL, Ackerman SE. The sociocultural dynamics of mass hysteria: a case study of social conflict in West Malaysia. Psychiatry. 1980;43:78–88.
71. Sham FM. Symptoms of hysteria among school-going adolescents in Malaysia: a conceptual study from the perspective of Islamic psychology. J Soc Sci Hum Pertanika. 2016;24(2):855–71.
72. Skeat WW. Malay magic. London: Macmillan; 1900.
73. Endicott K. An analysis of Malay magic. Oxford: Clarendon; 1970.
74. Gimlette J, Desmond J. Malay poisons and charm cures. London: Oxford University Press; 1915.
75. Fainting spells making school nervous. Oshkosh Daily Northwestern (WI). 10 Apr 1976. p. 1.
76. Explanation sought for teen-age fainting spells. Stevens Point Daily Journal [WI]. 10 Apr 1976. p. 11.
77. Fainting probe continues. Mobile Register (Mobile, AL). 11 Apr 1976. p. 18.
78. Fainting spells disrupt school, Kansas City Star (MO). 10 Apr 1976. p. 8.
79. Massad CM, Hubbard M, Newston D. Selective perception of events. J Exp Soc Psychol. 1978;15:513–32.

80. Jacobs N. The phantom slasher of Taipei: mass hysteria in a non-western society. Soc Probl. 1965;12:318–28.
81. 1954: Montreal slasher a myth?: in our pages: 100, 75 and 50 years ago. The New York Times. 30 Jan 2004.
82. Griffin E. Fight hysteria over Montreal leg slashings. The Chicago Tribune. 3 Jan 1954. p. 3.
83. Kumar L. DIG says 'shoot at monkeyman' as panic spreads. The Times of India. 14 May 2001.
84. Fathers M. Monkey man attack! simian assailant sweeps parts of New Delhi – anxious populace is gripped by terror. Time Asia. 28 May 2001;157.
85. Pregnant woman dies trying to escape as monkey-man panic grips India. Irish Examiner (Cork). 17 May 2001.
86. 'Monkey' gives Delhi claws for alarm. The Australian (NSW). 17 May 2001.
87. Sullivan M. Analysis: monkey man attacks in New Delhi. Morning Edition of American National Public Radio. 17 May 2001.
88. Ellis M. Find monkey man. City in terror after attacks by beast. Daily Record (Glasgow, Scotland). 17 May 2001. p. 29.
89. Harding L. Monkey man causes panic across Delhi. The Guardian. 18 May 2001. p. 12.
90. Pandey P. Cops step up hunt as panic spreads. The Hindu. 17 May 2001.
91. Maiti P. India's monkey man and the politics of mass hysteria. Skept Inq. 2001;25(5):8–9. See p. 9.
92. Bartholomew RE. Monkey man delusion sweeps India. The Skeptic Magazine (Altadena, CA). 2001;9(1):13.
93. Verma SK, Srivastava DK. A study on mass hysteria (monkey men?) victims in East Delhi. Indian J Med Sci. 2003;57(8):355–60.
94. Barber JW. Connecticut historical collections, containing a general collection of interesting facts traditions, biographical sketches, anecdotes, &c., relating to the history and antiquities of every town in Connecticut, with geographical descriptions. New Haven: John W. Barber; 1836. p. 446.
95. Robillard R. Windham and Williamantic. Charleston: Arcadia; 2005. p. 12.

A Short History of Spider, Insect, and Worm Scares

9

[U]nder certain conditions men respond as powerfully to fictions as they do to realities, and that in many cases they help to create the very fictions to which they respond.

–Walter Lippmann [1]

The 'sonic attack' saga in Cuba is not the first time that insects and other creepy crawlies have been implicated in triggering psychogenic episodes and social panics. Throughout history, spiders, insects and even worms have played a starring role. In this chapter, we will examine several examples. These are not just a series of colorful stories; they offer important insights into the events in Cuba, why it happened and when it happened. For instance, in Havana, crickets and cicadas blend into their natural surroundings and make strange noises that can be difficult to identify. Their presence, in conjunction with a stressful work environment and a history of surveillance and harassment of American diplomats, were instrumental in incubating the sonic attack hypothesis during the pivotal early stages. These tiny creatures make ideal subjects for social panics because there is a certain mystery about them and their alien appearance, and many become active under the cover of darkness. As a result, they have been the subject of Grade B movies featuring giant, menacing mutants that threaten human survival [2].

We begin our survey with Tarantism – a condition characterized by the uncontrollable urge to dance after being bitten by a tarantula spider. Tarantism has fascinated scholars for centuries. As noted in Chap. 5, episodes were concentrated in what is now southern Italy and were recorded as early as the thirteenth century. Widespread seasonal outbreaks persisted throughout Southern Europe, peaking in the seventeenth century, then rapidly declining. Tarantism was primarily confined to the height of the hot, dry months of July and August. Medical historian Henry Sigerist outlines the characteristic features: "People, asleep or awake, would suddenly jump up, feeling an acute pain like the sting of a bee. Some saw the spider, others did not, but they knew that it must be the tarantula. They ran out of the house into the street, to the marketplace dancing in great excitement. Soon they were joined by others who like

© Springer Nature Switzerland AG 2020
R. W. Baloh, R. E. Bartholomew, *Havana Syndrome*,
https://doi.org/10.1007/978-3-030-40746-9_9

them had just been bitten, or by people who had been stung in previous years, for the disease was never quite cured. The poison remained in the body and was reactivated every year by the heat of summer." He observed that the only effective remedies were music and dancing, and it was popularly believed that people would die if music was not available [3]. Those stricken were referred to as *tarantate*. Episodes are classified as a form of mass psychogenic illness as the condition was often contagious: for the appearance of one victim would commonly trigger symptoms in others [4]. In his review of the literature on Tarantism, neurologist Douglas Lanska concludes that there were multiple causes including psychogenic illness, ritualized behavior, and in some cases malingering [5]. In her study of ritualized behaviors inducing ecstasy, rapture, and trance-like states, Jerri Daboo views Tarantism as a regional idiom and means of coping, but often with a strong psychogenic component [6]. As medieval historian Peregrine Horden observes, "the spider's symbolism is more potent than its bite…. We are dealing with a culture-bound syndrome, or folk illness; with social and psychological 'poisoning' rather than a biological threat" [7]. Tarantism appears to be an interesting example of both the placebo and nocebo effect.

The ritualistic nature of cases is evident. As historian Jean Russell writes: "The dancers followed a set pattern and would begin dancing at sunrise, stop at midday, and go to bed and sweat, then have a bath and continue dancing until evening, when they would go to bed for another sweat, then rise for a light meal, and return to bed for the night. After 12 hours of dancing, even though they were exhausted, they became stronger and more agile. This ritual went on for four or five days, and in some cases weeks. The taranti acted like drunken people, remembering nothing afterwards. Some did this annually for as long as thirty years" [8]. Symptoms included headaches, fainting, breathing difficulties, chest pain, vomiting, trembling, twitching, excessive thirst, appetite loss, giddiness, general aches and pains, and hallucinations. These complaints parallel contemporary episodes of mass psychogenic illness in addition to the expected physical consequences from extended periods of exhaustive physical activity and alcohol consumption. The following is an eyewitness account involving a man in Southern Italy.

> I remember travelling together with some acquaintances in the wide, uneconomical regions which were drying out under the scorching sun. We heard the sound of drums, whistles and flutes in all the towns and villages and upon inquiring as to the meaning of it we were informed that in these regions it was a means of healing the people bitten by the tarantula. Then we went to a village and saw a young man affected by this disease. He seemed to have become insane, singing absentmindedly to the beat of a drum, while his arms and legs and the entire body moved in beat with the music. It was obvious that the sound of the drums pleased him and lessened his pain and he started to listen more and more to the instrument. Gradually his movements became more lively and finally he started to dance. It could appear to someone as being humorous and ridiculous but when the drummer stopped to play for a short period of time, the patient suddenly seemed to go numb, lose his senses and faint. However, as soon as the sound of drums could be heard again, the patient regained his strength and started to dance with more vigour than before. [8, p 405]

While 'victims' often claimed that a sore or swelling was the result of a tarantula bite, these assertions were difficult to verify as the bite was similar to other insects. Early observers theorized that a single bite from a venomous species of tarantula indigenous only to the 'boot' region of southern Italy, was responsible for Tarantism symptoms. However, as Sigerist observes: "The same tarantula shipped to other parts of the country seemed to lose most of its venom, and what remained acted differently" [3, p 221]. While the bite of *Latrodectus tarantula* can produce psychoactive effects, it is very slow moving, non-aggressive, and only in rare cases have victims experienced symptoms such as twitching, weakness, nausea and muscle pain. These symptoms are temporary and cannot account for the range or duration of Tarantism complaints. Furthermore, the identical species of spider is found across the world including the United States [9]. The species most commonly associated with tarantism, *Lycosa tarantula* – the Wolf Spider, is ferocious in appearance and has a painful bite, yet the symptoms are minor and typified by localized pain and itching [9, p 149]. The effects of its bite does not even remotely resemble Tarantism. It is doubtful that any species of spider or insect was responsible for 'attacks' as most participants did not even claim to have been bitten and would only participate in episodes at designated times. Some victims claim to have been possessed by the spider's 'spirit.'[10] Many bouts of Tarantism in Apulia were attributed to the bite of a scorpion [8], and while spider and tarantula bites, either real or perceived, were the most common means of 'infection,' an array of biting insects including ants were also blamed for triggering cases [6, p 4] The most common curative tunes were variants of the tarantella – an up-tempo dance which increases in intensity and is named after the Italian city of Taranto.

There is a histrionic component to Tarantism including the acting out of proscribed acts, often of a sexual nature. The diagnosis allows the victim to avoid the attribution of blame by claiming they had been under the influence of the tarantism spirit or venom. The dancing commonly endures for days, even weeks, in an intermittent fashion, until the victims proclaimed that they were 'cured,' only to relapse during subsequent summers. Some 'victims' claimed to be affected by merely brushing against the spider or scorpion or being in close proximity to those who had been bitten. Others were afflicted each summer upon hearing the strains of music being played as a cure for others who had been affected [9, pp 133–34]. The structure of the reactions appears to owe its origins to ancient Greek rituals which functioned as a cathartic reaction to pent-up stress. For over 1000 years prior to the first recorded incidents, followers of Pythagoras spread similar beliefs about the healing benefits of music, across what is now the Apulia region [11]. Remnants of Tarantism survive today in parts of Italy and take the form of festivals and cultural activities [12]. They illustrate the power of belief and the importance of tradition and ritual in shaping behaviors. It did not appear overnight but evolved slowly over time.

A modern-day outbreak of psychogenic symptoms involving spiders took place in Europe. Between late July and early August 2006, during a slow news period, a series of media reports appeared warning of the threat posed by *Cheiracanthium Punctorium* – the Yellow Sac Spider, including mild nausea and headaches. Each year, many Austrians are bitten by the spider, but in the wake of heightened media reporting about the insect's habits and sting, before long an influx of patients began presenting at emergency rooms and doctor's offices complaining of nausea and headaches, under the mistaken belief that they too had been bitten [13]. The Health Minister was forced to issue a statement calling for calm, noting that the spider's sting, while uncomfortable, was not life-threatening. In 1 day alone, 190 people flocked to the main hospital in the city of Linz with bite symptoms; doctors had excluded all but 8 as possible encounters with the spider [14].

The 'June Bug' Scare

A study of imaginary bug bites and mass suggestion took place during the summer of 1962. A textile Mill in Spartanburg, South Carolina was the scene of intense media scrutiny after 62 workers −59 women and 3 men reported symptoms that were attributed to mysterious insect bites. The local six o'clock TV news broke the story to the public, reporting that it was believed "that some kind of insect was in the shipment of cloth that arrived from England at the plant today. And at the moment the bug is blamed for the outbreak of sickness." The mill had a workforce of 965, meaning that about 6.5% were affected – over 95% female. That night, the same broadcast stated that according to a company employee, "the small insect attacks the skin, the bites leaving a wound similar to a gnat bite. In about 20 minutes the victim is struck with severe nausea." Within a couple of days, nine workers were admitted to the local hospital for treatment, while two more received emergency room treatment [15]. Complaints included fainting, headache, nausea, dizziness, disorientation, rashes, and fatigue [15, p 6]. Nineteen of the workers told of "almost fainting," while eight reported a feeling of general anxiety [16]. After a search of the premises, the only biting insect that was uncovered in the building was a chicken mite, which was incapable of producing the reported symptoms [16]. The Center for Disease Control investigated the outbreak along with an entomologist. A few days later, after the plant had been fumigated, the episode subsided. As one exterminator remarked: "Whatever has been here ain't here now" [15, p 7].

A sociological study of the episode was conducted by Alan Kerckhoff and Kurt Back of Duke University and Norman Miller of the University of Chicago. They concluded that the symptoms and belief in the 'bug' began in employees who were socially isolated, then spread quickly through social networks. The rate of spread was "a function of the fact that, as more cases appear, the behavior becomes increasingly legitimized – increasingly accepted according to an evolving generalized belief in the group involved." While 'outsiders' were slower to accept the bug's existence, as more and more workers exhibited symptoms, "the sheer size of the affected category makes the credibility of the phenomenon greater. We thus find that ultimately 'everyone' believes in 'the bug' … and cases begin to occur throughout the population. It thus becomes a 'crowd response'" [17]. Near the end of the episode, the *Charleston News and Courier* reported on the conclusion by experts that outbreak was psychogenic in origin.

Spartanburg (AP) – It's a mite's bite.
   Dr. J.C. Hedden Jr., county health officer, said Saturday that a report from the U.S. Public Health Service in Atlanta turned up a tiny mite labeled as a bird mite.

The little bug was picked up Friday by Health officials who vacuumed areas of the Butte Knitting Co. sewing room in an effort to find the culprit responsible in some way for the recent rash of illnesses at the plant....

The physician described it as a trigger setting off imagined sicknesses which literally become genuine illness....

The baffling part of the cases for attending physicians was that in many of the cases no sign of a bite could be detected.

Nausea, cramps, and numbness were symptoms of many of the patients. [18]

The outbreak could be traced to an incident involving a 22-year-old female worker who told her colleagues that she *may* have been bitten by an insect, before fainting. It was later revealed that the woman had a history of fainting. She had experienced no less than five episodes over the previous year. Three days later another worker reported that she too had recently been bitten by a mysterious bug, after which "she felt like a balloon ready to burst." [16, p 351] Later the same day, a third employee fainted, a women who had been under a physician's care for anxiety [16]. Later that day, a fourth plant worker sought medical aid after feeling a sensation like a crawling insect on her leg, before feeling faint. Researchers in the field of mass psychogenic illness often observe that in outbreaks at workplaces, those affected tend to be under greater stress than their co-workers, such as having tedious, repetitive jobs or poor relations with management. Kerckhoff and Back found that 95% of those affected by the 'June Bug' were women working in the dressmaking departments, who were more likely to accept the existence of an insect or other physical cause for the outbreak. They were more than twice as likely to be the sole income-earner, over 60% more likely to have worked overtime to three times per week, and five and a half times more likely to have been divorced, factors that may have increased their stress levels [19].

Bug Scares

South Africa has been the scene of several insect scares that have been blamed for the appearance of itching and rash, only to have been deemed psychogenic after no offending creatures were found. In mid-February 2000, students in 14 schools in the Free State Province of South Africa, deluged hospitals and clinics after an "itching phenomenon" swept through the region. Insects were seen as the most likely cause, although some residents were convinced that it was witchcraft. Most of the 1500 pupils affected were young girls [20]. During a 2-week period in February 2002, a similar outbreak of itching and rash swept across several schools in the Heidedal and Mangaung regions of South Africa. The symptoms were widely attributed to insect bites and affected 1400 mostly female students. Bug specialists were called in and scoured the buildings. Several book lice were found, but they were ever-present and common in local homes and factories. Based on the symptoms, entomologists focused their attention on a second suspect: an infection caused by itch mites, but none of the mites were found. The itching began soon after the students would enter the school grounds, only to subside when they returned home. Many of the students developed open sores from vigorous scratching. Methods of obtaining relief included rubbing the itchy part against walls, the use of scrubbing brushes, pens, rulers and stones. Other symptoms were headaches, dizziness, over-breathing, and chest tightness. Some were administered oxygen, no doubt stoking anxieties that were already high in the wake of rumors that two students had died from the itching. As is typical in cases of mass psychogenic illness, the symptoms were spread by line of sight after watching other students scratching. The outbreak subsided after the schools were closed and fumigated. Even though no insects were implicated in the episode, the highly publicized event of spraying the schools with insecticide and declaring them safe for use, would have convinced students that even if book and itch mites were responsible, they would have been dead by the time school reopened. An investigation by the Health Department and researchers at the University of the Free State concluded that the outbreak resulted from mass suggestion [21].

Another insect scare took place in September 2000, when a mysterious outbreak of itching, rash, and welts broke out at the Saxe Gotha Elementary School in Red Bank, South Carolina. The immediate suspicion was on bug bites, but the psychological element was quickly suspected by the unusual pattern of those affected, appearing most mornings soon after the students arrived at school but disappearing by lunchtime. As one parent observed: "It doesn't make any sense." Curiously, only students in Mrs. Steele's class were affected. Of her 18 pupils, 17 came down with the bumps and rash. The symptoms continued even after Mrs. Steele moved to a different classroom, and they went away when they were at home [22, 23].

> Itching a Mystery to S.C. School Officials
> COLUMBIA, S.C. (AP) – They've cleaned, fumigated, researched and even moved, but nearly every morning Carolyne Steele's second-grade class itches.
> Its been three months and officials still don't know why 17 of the 18 students in her room at Saxe Gotha Elementary…break out in a rash that disappears by lunch. ….
> The problem first appeared in mid-September. Steele and other adults thought it was caused by insect bites.
> The school called an exterminator and conducted careful searches to rule out lice and rabies. The custodial staff stepped up its cleaning of Steele's room. The air conditioner was checked. [24]

In January, health officials concluded that the episode was psychogenic, with State Health Director Linda Bell remarking that the evidence "strongly suggests they are susceptible to the power of suggestion from their classmates." However, the school principal rejected the idea, which is also a common reaction to cases of psychogenic illness [25]. A search of historical newspaper archives reveals similar cases that are often labeled as 'mystery illnesses' that eventually disappear.

Social Panics: From Kissing Bugs to Cabbage Worms

It is important to understand that when psychiatrists use the term delusion, it typically refers to an array of conditions in people who are suffering from psychosis and have difficulty distinguishing fantasy from reality. They may experience hallucinations or think they are being watched. Psychotic delusions include conditions such as schizophrenia. However, sociologists use the term to describe the spontaneous spread of false beliefs within a given population of overwhelmingly normal, healthy people. At first glance, these accounts may appear somewhat tangential and off-topic, but as we will show, they are directly related to what happened in Cuba – and there are important commonalities. They demonstrate how social delusions, with or without accompanying health complaints, never occur in a vacuum; each is couched in unique social, cultural and political contexts that people found plausible. In the case of the Great Kissing Bug Scare, it was a single journalist who was responsible for igniting fear of an insect that had previously been perceived as relatively harmless. In the case of the Texas earthworm hoax, while it may seem inconceivable that many residents of Laredo believed that a massive earthworm carcass was on a major Interstate Highway, many citizens believed it because of the local belief in the existence of giant earthworms which have a longstanding tradition in Central and South America. Likewise, the 'sonic attack' was incubated in an atmosphere of long held suspicion and fear of Cuban operatives surveilling US Embassy staff in Havana. This history shaped the early interpretation of the sounds and symptoms that were being reported, and was assumed to have been caused by some type of surveillance or harassment. If the same sounds and symptoms had been reported by US Embassy staff in France or the United Kingdom, those involved would likely not have given it a second thought. They would have been interpreted as mundane sounds and unrelated symptoms. Talk of a sonic weapon would have been deemed absurd.

During the late nineteenth century, an influx of kissing bug bites were recorded in the United States. The episode is an example of a social delusion as people began to redefine events and circumstance as kissing bug-related. Kissing bugs refer to an array of insect species that suck blood from mammals. They get their name from their habit of piercing the skin of sleeping victims, often on the face, and occasionally on the lips. During the summer of 1899, a wave of kissing bug 'attacks' were reported across the United States. The bug has a reputation for being deadly in parts of Latin America, where it is notorious for spreading Chagas disease. However, the species of kissing bugs in the US rarely infect humans, and the chance of contracting Chagas is extremely low. The insect's bad image and sensational journalism contributed to the scare.

The kissing bug panic began with the publication of an article written by *Washington Post* police reporter James McElhone. In mid-June 1899, he wrote about a spike in the number of patients seeking treatment. On June 20, McElhone published a dramatic, speculative story about the dangers of kissing bugs, frightening readers with claims that people had been "badly poisoned." Ominously, he issued a warning that the worst may be yet to come, writing that it "threatens to become something like a plague" [26]. The headline read: "Bite of a Strange Bug. Several Patients Have Appeared at the Hospitals Very Badly Poisoned." The tone of the story would have made many readers anxious. "Look out for the new bug. It is an insidious insect that bites without causing pain and escapes unnoticed. But afterward the place it has bitten swells to ten times its normal size. The Emergency Hospital has had several victims of this insect lately and the number is increasing. Application for treatment by other victims are being made at other hospitals, and the matter threatens to become something like a plague. None of those who have been bitten saw the insect whose sting proves so disastrous. One old negro went to sleep and woke up to find both his eyes nearly closed by the swelling from his nose and cheeks, where the insect had alighted. The lips seems to be the favored point of attack." He then made the curious comment that no one who had been bitten had actually seen the insect [26].

Other papers in the nation's capital quickly followed suit, reporting on the outbreak of kissing bug attacks. Before long, newspapers across the county were reporting on the threat. Not surprisingly, accounts of kissing bug attacks began pouring in across the country as citizens were on the lookout for the dreaded bug or any insect that remotely resembled it [27]. Soon people began attributing any insect bite, swelling or discomfort on or near their face as the work of the kissing bug. The Chief of Entomology for the US Department of Agriculture in Washington D.C., Leland Howard, described the panic as a "*newspaper* epidemic, for every insect bite where the biter was not at once recognized was attributed to the popular and somewhat mysterious creature" [27, p 34]. The chief suspect in many newspaper accounts was *Melanolestes picipes*, despite its previous good reputation among entomologists. An insect expert wrote in *Scientific American* that kissing bugs were no more common during the summer of 1899 than any other year, and they were no more harmful [28].

Dozens of specimens from suspected attacks from across the country were sent to bug specialists at the Philadelphia Academy of Natural Sciences. No less than 21 different species were identified including everything from the common housefly to bees, beetles – even a butterfly. Not a single kissing bug was among them [29]. In New York, scores of insects were sent to the State entomologist Dr. E.P. Felt for identification. "All thus far received have proved to be harmless insects, lacking poisonous attachments." Felt cautioned readers that it was rare for a kissing bug to land on someone's lips, noting that the bug was passive, only attacking in self-defense. "This bug will not steal into a room and pounce upon a sleeping victim. To be stung, a person must go into its vicinity and cause it harm" [30].

A contributing factor in the scare was the menacing appearance of *Melanolestes picipes,* which looked guilty. In Chicago, when a man spotted a kissing bug, he captured it as a precaution despite it having made no attempt to bite anyone. "The bug is a strange looking insect and appears to deserve all the mean things that have been said of him. It…has a short, strong beak, with a point as sharp as that of a mosquito. Its color is nearly black… [31]. As the scare grew, press accounts of kissing bug 'attacks' grew increasingly sensational [28]. One report from a woman in Chicago resembled a vampire attack from a horror movie as it was claimed: "The marks of two small incisors could be seen" [32]. In Philadelphia, the presence of what was thought to have been a kissing bug on a street car was met with shrieks and screams as several women were on the verge of leaping off the carriage [33].

The scare intensified in mid-July after several deaths were attributed to the insect, each under dubious circumstances. A coroner in Chicago linked the death of Mary Steger to the bug. The attending physician, Dr. George Illingworth, wrote that "Mrs. Steger was stung 6 days before her death… She distinctly remembered having been stung, but did not succeed in capturing the bug. The sting was on the upper lip, and the mark was plainly perceptible, even before the face swelled." But while her death certificate officially stated that the cause of death was "the sting of a kissing bug," making headlines across the country, tonsillitis was listed as a contributing cause. The accuracy of the autopsy was called into question because by the time the body was examined, it had already been embalmed, making it difficult to determine the exact cause of death [34]. In Trenton, New Jersey, when a 2-year-old toddler suddenly died under mysterious circumstances, the attending doctor linked the bug to the death after finding an ambiguous "red spot" on the girl's leg [35]. Headlines of kissing bug deaths would have no doubt alarmed many citizens. On July 15, the front page of the *Evansville Journal* in Indiana proclaimed: "Young Woman Dead and Two Men Suffering."

> WATERLOO, IA., July 14. – Mary Vaughn, a young woman of Cedar Falls, died last night from a bite on her lip from a bug. It is supposed to be from a 'Kissing Bug.' The young woman was bitten a week ago. Her face and head swelled so they were unrecognizable…
>
> BEDFORD, IND. July 14. – The kissing bug has made its appearance in this city, having begun its work last night on Newton Anderson, whose lip to-day is swollen out of all shape. It is in such a condition that Mr. Anderson can scarcely talk and can partake only of liquid. Physicians apprehend no danger and say the swelling will go down in a day or two.
>
> WARSAW, IND., July 14 – The kissing bug has made its appearance in this city, when John Breeding, a resident of this place, woke up this morning his face was alarmingly swollen. Doctors were summoned and did everything in their power to relieve the sufferer, who is now thought to be out of danger. The doctors say that Breeding was the victim of the bug commonly known as the kissing bug, and it was only prompt remedial application that saved him. [36]

Some newspaper editors were rightly dubious of the sudden flurry of kissing bug 'attacks' and recognized the scare for what it was. In Rockford, Illinois, the *Register-Gazette* reported that several local girls had "been on the streets every night in the hope of meeting a kissing bug [37]. The editor of the San Francisco *Call*, John McNaught, aptly summed up the scare when he wrote: "The prevailing sputter and flurry over the kissing bug is a striking illustration of the old proverb, 'We always see what we look for.'" Alluding to the power of the press to artificially drum up excitement, and the proclivity of the human imagination to create 'monsters' when none exist, he made a conspicuous observation that many citizens had failed to recognize. He observed how odd and unusual the outbreak was, for "all at once, the creature appears simultaneously all over the United States; and every community has its thrilling tale to tell of the terrors of the creature's kiss" [38]. This state of affairs was reinforced by the official entomologist for the state of New Jersey, Professor John B. Smith, who noted that the hoop-la surrounding the insect, was just that. "I have been bitten by them many a time," he said, and if anyone will bring me a live kissing bug I will let it sting to its heart's content. We are simply going through a craze like the one we had when spider bites were popular. Everybody who was bitten by any kind of an insect was bitten by a spider. The same is true now." He observed that kissing bugs feed on caterpillars and other insects, and "sometimes convey poisons, but the insect is no more numerous or dangerous now than it ever was" [39].

The Seattle Windshield Pitting 'Epidemic'

Sand fleas played a role in another American social delusion, although no psychogenic symptoms were recorded. Known to sociologists as 'The Seattle Windshield Pitting Epidemic,' and discussed in Chap. 1, the episode began in late March 1954, when tiny pockmarks were noticed on windshields in the vicinity of Bellingham, Washington. Initially thought to have been the work of vandals with BB-guns, by mid-April, reports of the mysterious pitting had reached all the way to Seattle amid a flurry of newspaper accounts speculating as to the cause. One hypothesis held that sand flea eggs were responsible for the marks and the tiny creatures were hatching in the glass [40]. A Centralia, Washington man, Jack Scherer, elaborated on the hypothesis. "What actually has happened is that in securing the sand for the windshield glass, sand flea eggs also were gathered. The eggs remained in the glass and, with the approach of warm weather, the windshields warmed up, the eggs hatched and the fleas have to chip the glass to get out" [41]. However, it would have been impossible for the fleas to have survived the making of the glass which occurs at high temperatures, and then to have escaped their glass enclosure. By April 15, the Mayor of Seattle contacted President Dwight Eisenhower, asking for emergency assistance in solving the mystery. A group of scientists at the University of Washington concluded that the windshield marks had always been there, but in the wake of media publicity about the 'mysterious pits,' residents began to look at instead of through their windshields [42, 43].

The American Cabbage Worm Panic

The Great Cabbage Worm Scare waxed and waned during the latter nineteenth and early twentieth centuries and is a classic example of a rumor and an urban legend that was so firmly and widely believed, that it was latched onto by newspaper reporters across the country and presented as fact. Urban legends are 'foaf tales' – friend of a friend tales that are founded on hearsay and passed on as true by the teller. During autumn 1903, alarming newspaper accounts began to appear of people having been poisoned after eating cooked cabbage that contained a poisonous worm. Many reported deaths were attributed to these nefarious creatures sometimes dubbed 'cabbage snakes.' *The Evening News* of San Jose, California proclaimed: "Poisoned by Cabbage." It stated: "Great loss of life is reported in the counties of Northeast Georgia, due to eating cabbage saturated with poison by a strange worm. During the past few weeks persons coming here from White, Townes, Union, Dawson, Forsythe and other counties surrounding them have reported scores of deaths from this cause… At first the mysterious deaths were not understood and all occurred after the eating of cabbage" [44]. In October, the *Atlanta Constitution* reported that a farmer in White County Georgia was gathering cabbage when he discovered a thread-like worm in a head. "He says it licked its tongue out like a snake when he touched the leaf it was on, and that it was shaped very much like a snake… He became alarmed and to satisfy himself as to what it was he sent it to the state chemist for analysis to see whether or not it was poisonous. The state chemist analyzed it and reported that there was enough poison in the thing to kill fifteen persons" [45]. Suspiciously, and in classic urban legend fashion, neither the name of the farmer nor the chemist involved were identified. The account was later discredited. In fact, there is no evidence of a single death or illness having been caused by eating cabbage worms [46].

The scare was even reported in the *New York Times*. In August 1904, it said that many people had become ill after "eating cabbage in which snakes had been boiled have attracted wide attention in various parts of Tennessee, and the latest is the Morilton family, at Tullahoma, where several people are ill." As a result of the scare, people were said to have been carefully searching their vegetables for the creatures. "Many people have quit eating cabbages, and the result is that with the biggest crop ever produced in the State, they are selling at 20 cents a barrel, while in the small towns one cannot give them away, and they are being fed to live stock" [47]. Cabbage snakes were also implicated in the mysterious deaths of animals. One man in Grand River, Iowa, claimed he fed one of the snakes to his cat, which promptly dropped dead [48].

In 1904, different states began to address the reports in an effort to refute them. For instance, biologist Gerald McCarthy wrote in the bulletin of the North Carolina Agriculture Department, that the "snake" was harmless. He equated the scare to the annual sea serpent 'silly season,' being replaced "by a land serpent which has located in the western part of North Carolina, where it has taken to frightening the owners of cabbage patches" [49]. He noted that the many reported deaths from the creature were both unfounded and ridiculous. He said that the creatures contained no venom, and if one were to eat cabbage harboring the worm, the consequences would be far greater to the worm than the human [49].

In January 1905, a Des Moines, Iowa wholesale produce merchant J. W. Brown expressed extreme frustration over the spread of the Cabbage Snake myth, proclaiming: "Five million dollars paid for a lie." It was reported that cabbage heads were rotting in produce cellars across Des Moines as residents were fearful of eating them in the wake of the rumors. The losses were estimated at upwards of $10,000, while the nationwide losses were placed at five million [50]. By May 1905, the US Agriculture Department was so concerned by the impact from the scare that it issued a special report that was published in many newspapers, exposing the myth of the cabbage snake. When it was reissued again in 1908, it again prompted a salvo of skeptical articles. In his 1908 report to the US Department of Agriculture, entomologist F. H. Chittenden concluded that the scare was triggered by people misidentifying the cabbage hair-worm, which was not toxic. They are white worms about the thickness of horse hair. He blamed the scare on poor journalism as the many press reports about the dreaded cabbage snake appear to have been based on an existing urban legend and hearsay, with the journalists and local correspondents never bothering to check the claims firsthand in order to verify them. Chittenden noted that while the length of the hair-worm could vary from 2 to 9 inches, and had the thickness of horsehair, some press reports claimed that the worm or snake was 9 feet long! "The imagination of newspaper writers as to color runs riot through 'green, white, light red, olive green, and yellow,'" he said [46, p 2]

The editor of *The Citizen* newspaper in Berea, Kentucky, Silas Mason, concurred with Chittenden's assessment, placing much of the blame for the scare on his newspaper colleagues. He hypothesized that the origin of the story came from a young reporter trying "to fill up space" on a slow news day. "Somebody's family had been sick, as is not uncommon in days of hot weather and green apples and garden truck (bartering). Somebody said he thought it was cabbage they had eaten hurt them. The news hunter had his pencil good and sharp and it was a dull day for news so he thought to try a bit of fiction. To say that Old Man Blank's three children and the hired girl had cholera morbus would be only a small item and common place. To blame boiled cabbage for it would not add much, but here the genius of the fellow came to the surface; the power of invention" [51].

Chittenden observed that while the worm was not in the least bit injurious to health, the consequences of the stories did have significant effects, resulting in the plummeting financial value of cabbage in some parts of the country. In sections of Illinois, both cabbage growers and purchasers were suffering financial hardship as farmers were letting their crop rot in the field. In Quinter, Kansas, cabbage shipped from Colorado was burned as a precaution. In Tennessee, an estimated 85% of the state's 1904 cabbage crop was reported lost. Missouri was also hard hit, where across several counties including Cheatham, Smith, Franklin, Bedford, and Coffee and other regions of the state, "hundreds of barrels of sauerkraut were destroyed through fear that the dreaded snake might be a part of the ingredients." At Columbia, Missouri, hundreds of dollars worth of cabbage was lost in the "snake scare," with gardeners claiming that they could not sell a single head [52]. *The Warsaw Daily Union* reported on an incident in nearby Illinois, involving a family of six that were allegedly wiped out after eating the snake [53]. This account appeared in numerous newspapers, yet when Chittenden checked with a local official, he could not confirm the story. Certainly, if a family had reportedly died from eating tainted cabbage, a prominent community figure would have been aware of it [46, p 4]. Worried residents from across the country mailed in specimens of suspected hair-worms to the US Agriculture Department's Bureau of Entomology. They received everything from caterpillars to moths and butterflies, even earthworms and fly larvae [46, p 5].

To allay widespread public fears over the poisonous nature of the hair-worm, Dr. Louis Leroy of Nashville, Tennessee, conducted experiments with both raw and cooked hair-worms by feeding them to cats, dogs, guinea pigs, rabbits, cows, and horses. None showed any harmful effect. He even considered the possibility that when the worms decompose and ferment in the cabbage, they may produce poisons. His analysis failed to find any cause for alarm [46, p 6]. As for the numerous reports of people experiencing stomach pain and vomiting after consuming cabbage later found to have been contaminated with the worms, in addition to the likelihood of some of these accounts having been rumors, Chittenden suggested the possibility of "mass hysteria" [46, p 4].

Like many papers, *The Ellensburgh Capital* in Washington State cited Chittenden's 1905 report and proclaimed: "Cabbage Snake Fake" [54]. The *Weekly Kentucky New Era* stated "Entirely Harmless. So Called Cabbage Worm a Well Meaning Reptile" [55]. While the scare waned dramatically with the warning by the

Department of Agriculture, it flared up again in the first half of 1908. In early January, the *Gainesville Sun* reported that Mrs. R. E. Dashiell of Orange Heights "came within a little of losing her life or the life of the entire family a day or two ago… and it was only by the merest chance that, while she was cleaning a head of cabbage for dinner," she discovered the creature. The reporter stated that the worm was "said to be almost deadly poison when cooked with a pot of cabbage" [56]. In March, the *Brownsville Daily Herald* in Texas reported that "the cabbage snake when boiled with cabbage is dangerous to the health" [57]. Concerned by the new wave of press reports spreading the myth, Agriculture Department officials released an updated bulletin on July 28 on the harmless nature of the creature. This, in turn, prompted a second wave of newspaper articles critical of the hair-worm being a harbinger of death.

Erroneous stories about the 'deadly' hair-worm continued to appear in the press in a sporadic fashion for years. In Kansas, the *Lawrence Daily Journal* of August 9, 1910, reported on the front page that "the dreaded 'cabbage snake' was discovered by Mrs. Lida Morris last Monday morning when she was preparing a head of cabbage for dinner. It is one of the first specimens of the rare and strange reptile ever seen in Sedgwick county, although 2 years ago several members of a family are said to have died after eating cabbage containing the snake" [58]. In October 1912, *The Champaign Democrat* in Urbana, Ohio, reported on a close call with "the reptile" in a six-gallon vat of sauerkraut, narrowly averting disaster [59]. Two months later, the same paper reported that years earlier, three soldiers had died near the Georgia-Tennessee border after eating cabbage snakes. Their source: a Spanish-American War veteran whose word they had taken [60]. In September 1922, the South Carolina-based *Spartanburg Herald* reported that consuming cabbage and sauerkraut were taboo following an incident near Greenwood when a specimen of cabbage snake "believed by some to cause instant death if eaten, had been captured and caged in a peanut butter jar here, where it is being watched with fearful interest by cabbage consumers. Some insist that to eat the thing means death by poisoning" [61]. As late as 1935, the 'snake' was identified in Florida. *The Sarasota Herald* reported that a small milk bottle was brought to the *Herald* office with a one-inch-long "cabbage snake" that the possessor claimed was "more poisonous than a rattle-snake" [62]. The press clearly played a major role in keeping the myth of the deadly cabbage worm alive for so long.

Earthworm!

Our final example of social delusions is the story of a giant earthworm in Laredo, Texas. In early March 1993, *The Morning Times of Laredo* published a fake news story about a 300-pound, 79-foot long worm that had supposedly been run over by a vehicle with its body lying on Interstate 35, blocking traffic. The story appeared on page 3A under the headline, "Agents recover huge carcass." The journalist who wrote the article, Carol Huang, was fired the same day the story appeared. She claimed that she had written the story as a joke and was shocked when the editor,

Tom Sanchez, put it in the paper. She told the *American Journalism Review*, "I knew right away I was in trouble" [63]. Aside from the bizarre claim, the account was presented in a credible fashion, complete with an interview with a scientist from Laredo State University who speculated that the creature may have mutated from the nearby Rio Grande River. According to the report, Laredo police and Border Patrol officers had converged on the site, wearing rubber gloves and assisting in the removal of the remains with the aid of two cranes and a large truck [63]. Local police received hundreds of calls from residents – many who drove to the scene in hopes of seeing the giant worm, and in the process, causing a traffic jam. The final paragraph of the article by reporter Carol Huang, led to the tie-up. She wrote: "Because federal environmental guidelines do not outline the proper disposal method for large, earthworm carcasses...authorities have left the creature in the Target store parking lot until Monday, when zoologists and EPA (Environmental Protection Agency) officials are expected to arrive from Washington" [63]. Even before the store had opened that morning, people were tapping on windows and asking employees if the worm was there. The Target parking lot soon became the focus of attention as curiosity seekers flocked to the scene. Border Patrol spokesman Alfonso Moreno said, "There was a lot of commotion, cars going in and out of there, looking for the worm." Huang would later observe that she never realized the extent to which "people read the newspaper and believe what they read" [63].

The earthworm hoax could not have occurred had it not been rendered plausible by the local culture. Laredo is situated on the US-Mexican border, and many residents hail from Central and South America, which are rife with tales of giant earthworm-like creatures. Just like many people believe in the existence of Bigfoot or the Loch Ness Monster, south of the border there is a widespread belief in giant worms that dwell in lakes and ponds. In Nicaragua they are known as *sierpe*; in other regions, they are referred to as *Surubin-Rei*. In Brazil they are the *minhocão* (literally 'giant earthworm'), and any mysterious trench or burrow may be attributed to their presence, as are sinkholes [52, 64–66]. Tales of these creatures may have inspired the popular 1990 film *Tremors*, where carnivorous earthworms dubbed Graboids terrorize a small Nevada town. The popularity of the film inspired several sequels.

Each of the scares outlined in this chapter are relevant to the events in Cuba as they highlight the power of belief. What they have in common is the key role of plausibility and the importance of historical context in incubating episodes. Whenever people accept the reality of anything, it can have real-world consequences, even if that belief is a figment of the human imagination. These incidents may seem trivial or humorous, but it is worth remembering that social realities can have serious ramifications. Claims by the State Department and other government officials, including Donald Trump, that American Embassy staff were deliberately targeted by a mysterious energy force and that the Cubans were involved, has resulted in serious repercussions for diplomatic ties with the island nation. It has stoked anger and mistrust in our Caribbean neighbor at a delicate time in our relations. It has also generated unnecessary fear and given rise to an array of conspiracy theories and a belief in the existence of a secret weapon that is capable of making people sick. And we cannot forget the Embassy staff, who are victims of a narrative that has no basis in fact but has had a powerful impact on the lives of the men and women who were serving as diplomats, along with their families.

References

1. Lippmann W. Public opinion. Mineola: Dover; 2004. p. 7.
2. Clay K. A mouth full of maggots, a review of the infested mind: why humans fear, loathe, and love insects. Bioscience. 2014;64(12):1189–91. https://doi.org/10.1093/biosci/biu161.
3. Sigerist HE. Civilization and disease. Ithaca: Cornell University Press; 1943. p. 218–9.
4. Bynum B. Discarded diagnoses: tarantism. Lancet. 2001;358:1736.
5. Lanska DJ. The dancing manias: psychogenic illness as a social phenomenon. In: Bogousslavsky J, editor. Neurologic-psychiatric syndromes in focus - part II: from psychiatry to neurology. Basel: Karger; 2018. p. 132–41.
6. Daboo J. Ritual, rapture and remorse: a study of tarantism and pizzica in Salento. New York: Peter Lang; 2010. p. 4.
7. Horden P, editor. Music as medicine: the history of music therapy since antiquity. Burlington: Ashgate; 2000. p. 250.
8. Russell JF. Tarantism. Med Hist. 1979;23:404–25. See p. 413.
9. Bartholomew RE. Exotic deviance: medicalizing cultural idioms–from strangeness to illness. Boulder: University Press of Colorado; 2000. p. 149.
10. Kearney C, Trull T. Abnormal psychology and life: a dimensional approach. Boston: Cengage Learning; 2018. p. 12–3.
11. Inglis B. A brief history of medicine. London: Weidenfeld; 1965. p. 66.
12. Ludtke K. Tarantism in contemporary Italy: the tarantula's dance reviewed and revived. In: Horden P, editor. Music as medicine. Burlington: Ashgate; 2000. p. 292–313.
13. Moore T. Did you hear? The Times (London). 7 Aug 2006. p. 2.
14. Maan N. Spider invasion creeping out Austrians. Associated Press. 3 Aug 2006.
15. Kerckhoff AC. Analyzing a case of mass psychogenic illness. In: Colligan M, Pennebaker J, Murphy L, editors. Mass psychogenic illness: a social psychological analysis. New York: Routledge; 2009. p. 5–20. See p. 6.
16. Champion F, Taylor R. Mass hysteria associated with insect bites. J S C Med Assoc. 1963;59:351–3. See p. 352.
17. Kerckhoff A, Back K, Miller N. Sociometric patterns in hysterical contagion. Sociometry. 1965;28:2–15. See p. 13.
18. Mite started Spartanburg mill furor. Charleston News and Courier (Charleston, SC). 24 Jun 1962. p. 45.
19. Kerckhoff A, Back K. The June bug: a study of hysterical contagion. New York: Appleton-Century-Crofts; 1968.
20. Mystery school itch 'caused by witches.' South African Press Association. 21 Feb 2000.
21. Rataemane S, Rataemane L, Mohlahle J. Mass hysteria among student learners at Mangaung schools in Bloemfontein, South Africa. Int J Psychosoc Rehabil. 2002;6:61–7.
22. Robinson B. Mysterious itching plagues Saxe Gotha. The State (Columbia, SC). 5 Dec 2000. p. 1.
23. Tests seek cause for second graders' itching. The State. 6 Dec 2000. p. 7.
24. Itching a mystery to S.C. school officials. Gaston Gazette (Gastonia, NC). 6 Dec 2000; Sect. 6:B.
25. Shannon King, Report says rash caused by power of suggestion. The State. 4 Jan 2000. p. 5.
26. McElhone J. Bite of a strange bug. The Washington Post. 20 Jun 1899.
27. Howard LO. Spider bites and 'kissing bugs.' Popular Science Monthly. 1899;56:31–42. See p. 34.
28. Murray-Aaron E. The kissing bug scare. Sci Am. 1899;81:54.
29. Editorial. Entomol News. 1899;10:205–6.

30. The kissing bug. The Brooklyn Eagle. 17 July 1899.
31. Captured a kissing bug. Fort Wayne Evening Sentinel (IN). 19 July 1899.
32. Weird tales of kissing bug. The Chicago Daily Tribune. 11 July 1899. p. 2.
33. A kissing bug panic. The Daily Advocate (Baton Rouge, LA). 9 Sept 1899. p. 3.
34. Cause of death a kissing bug. The San Francisco Call. 19 July 1899. p. 3.
35. Died of a kissing bug's bite. Naugatuck Daily News (Naugatuck, CT). 19 July 1899.
36. Young woman dead and two mend suffering. Evansville Journal (Evansville, IN). 15 July 1899. p. 1.
37. The kissing bug. The Chicago Tribune. 20 July 1899. p. 7.
38. McNaught J. Editorial variations. The San Francisco Call. 23 July 1899. p. 6.
39. Kissing bugs harmless. The Pacific Commercial Advertiser (Honolulu, HI). 22 Aug 1899. p. 4.
40. Hatching of sand fleas in glass suggested in windshield pocking; even FBI called into case. The Oregonian (Portland, OR). 25 Apr 1954. p. 17.
41. Gives reason for pitting. Sand fleas are doing damage. Daily Illinois State Journal (Springfield, IL). 22 Apr 1954. p. 14.
42. Medalia NZ, Larsen O. Diffusion and belief in a collective delusion. Sociological Review. 1958;23:180–6.
43. Berenbaum M. Insects and windshields – a crash course. Am Entomol. 2002;48(1):1–2.
44. Poisoned by cabbage. Was saturated with poison by a strange worm. The Evening News (San Jose, CA). 23 Oct 1903. p. 8.
45. Deadly poison causes dread. The Atlanta Constitution (GA). 22 Oct 1903. p. 1.
46. Chittenden FH. The cabbage hair-worm. Circular No. 62. United States Department of Agriculture Bureau of Entomology. 17 May 1905. In 1908, a revised edition was issued July 28 under the same title.
47. Boiled cabbage and snakes. The New York Times. 13 Aug 1904. p. 2.
48. Cabbage snakes in Iowa. Dubuque Daily Telegraph (IA). 17 Oct 1904. p. 8.
49. Cabbage snakes are but harmless little worms. Weekly Kentucky New Era. 18 Nov 1905. p. 4.
50. Cost of the cabbage snake. The Ithaca Democrat (NY). 26 Jan 1905. p. 4.
51. The cabbage snake. The Citizen (Berea, KY). 3 Aug 1905. p. 3.
52. Roe PG. Process in South Amerindian oral narratives. R Anthrop. 1982;9(3):269–85. See p. 272.
53. Ate poisoned cabbage. entire family of six, living near Siddell, Ill., dead as a result. Warsaw Daily Union (IN). 12 Dec 1904. p. 3.
54. Cabbage snake fake. The Ellensburgh Capital. 16 Aug 1905. p. 4.
55. Entirely harmless. Weekly Kentucky New Era. 16 June 1905. p. 3.
56. This lady found a cabbage snake. The Gainesville Sun. 6 Jan 1908. p. 5.
57. Untitled. Brownsville Daily Herald (TX). 19 Mar 1908. p. 2.
58. Cabbage snake. Lawrence Daily Journal (KS). 9 Aug 1910. p. 1.
59. Snake is found in cabbage head. poisonous variety had been chopped into sauer kraut. The Champaign Democrat (Urbana, OH). 8 Oct 1912. p. 2.
60. New menace has been found. The Champaign Democrat. 3 Dec 1912. p. 2.
61. Fearsome cabbage snake back again to frighten people. Spartanburg Herald (SC). 2 Sept 1922. p. 2.
62. 'Cabbage snake' is exhibited here. The Sarasota Herald (FL). 26 Apr 1935. p. 1.
63. Martinez Y. A long, tall Texas tale. Am Journal Rev. 1993;15(4):11.
64. Bane T. Encyclopedia of beasts and monsters in myth, legend and folklore. Jefferson: McFarland; 2016. p. 226.
65. de Saint-Hilaire MA. On the Minhocão of the Goyanes. Am J Sci. 1847;2(4):130–1.
66. Eberhart G. Mysterious creatures: a guide to cryptozoology. Santa Barbara: ABC-CLIO; 2002. p. 337–8.

State Terrorism Masquerading as Psychogenic Illness

10

The self-fulfilling prophecy is, in the beginning, a false definition of the situation evoking a new behavior which makes the originally false conception come true.

–Thomas K. Merton [1]

There are several cases where a foreign government was initially blamed for the appearance of mysterious symptoms similar to those in Havana, that after careful examination, were found to have been psychogenic in nature. In this chapter, we present examples of outbreaks that were purportedly launched by a hostile foreign power, with whom there had been longstanding political tension. Like the Cuban episode, each of our cases appeared amid rumors and media publicity that gave credence to the imaginary attack. *Many of these episodes included neurological symptoms*. It is noteworthy that the health complaints in Cuba did not appear suddenly, but gradually over months. They emerged in a group of people who knew they were being watched every minute of the day and night. They were in a hostile foreign country, and the stress from being constantly surveilled was relentless.

Pseudo-Poisonings in the Middle East

The West Bank is a piece of land that separates the neighboring countries of Israel and Jordan. It is one of the most hotly disputed territories in the world. The region was taken over by Israel after the June 1967 Arab-Israeli War in order to create a buffer zone between the two countries. Prior to this time, the area was overseen by Jordan. Since the war, the many Palestinians who live there refer to it as an occupied territory. The issue is an emotional one for many Palestinians who believe that their land has been unjustly taken from them. It has also been the site of many protests over the years and fierce anti-Israeli sentiments. It was within this tense atmosphere of suspicion and distrust that a strange illness broke out on the morning of March 21, 1983, at an all-girls' school in the West Bank town of Arrabah. A 17-year-old

© Springer Nature Switzerland AG 2020
R. W. Baloh, R. E. Bartholomew, *Havana Syndrome*,
https://doi.org/10.1007/978-3-030-40746-9_10

student began to complain of dizziness, headaches, blurry vision, and breathing problems [2]. Over the next hour or so, 10 of her classmates were stricken with similar symptoms after complaining of a bad smell resembling rotten eggs. Within a few hours, 15 more girls were taken ill, and by the end of the next day, 61 schoolgirls and 5 adults had been rushed to nearby hospitals. Many had fainted. The next day, the Israeli evening newspaper *Yedi'ot Abronot* reported on the outbreak, claiming that the girls were suffering from blindness, headaches, and abdominal pain as well as cyanosis, a bluish discoloration of their arms and legs due to the lack of oxygen [3]. This report was alarming, sensational, and contained several erroneous claims. The journalist who wrote the story described the events in melodramatic fashion and suggested poison gas as the cause. Two girls were said to have been suffering from "complete blindness," and breathing problems that were so severe they needed to be transferred to an Israeli hospital in Affula. In reality, they were experiencing blurred vision and over-breathing. The claims of cyanosis were never verified, and there was no evidence of an attack. The appearance of this report, within a backdrop of long-held suspicion and animosity between Israelis and Palestinians in the West Bank, provided the spark for a series of escalating events that would follow. Before the episode would end 2 weeks later, nearly a thousand mostly Arab schoolgirls had succumbed to the sickness.

On March 26, 246 girls and staff in six schools in the town of Jenin and two neighboring villages developed similar symptoms to those in the Arrabah 'attack.' On this occasion, another Israeli evening newspaper, *Ma'Ariv,* ran a story with the headline "THE MYSTERIOUS POISONING GOES ON: 56 HIGH SCHOOL GIRLS IN JENIN POISONED" [3, p 835]. The article stated that 29 girls from Jenin High School were admitted to hospital in the morning and an additional 27 throughout the day with dizziness, difficulty breathing and cyanosis. It said that the source of the "poisoning" was unknown. Amid the growing crisis, Israeli psychiatrist Dr. Albert Hefez was asked to investigate. He later reported the chaotic scene when he arrived at the Jenin Hospital, a small town facility with about 100 beds. A rather large entry reception hall served as a staging area for emergency admissions during the crisis. Local police guarded the entrance to the hall. Upon entering, Dr. Hefez observed many people who did not belong to the hospital staff including foreign newspaper reporters interviewing staff and patients. "The situation in this improvised emergency room suddenly became dramatic when a teen-age Arab girl on a stretcher was brought into the hospital accompanied by her mother. She was immediately surrounded by a group of medical and paramedical workers, who pushed the mother aside. An oxygen mask was forcibly applied to the girl's face, and an intramuscular injection was administered almost simultaneously. The mother kept at a distance from her daughter, apparently intimidated and helpless" [3, p 836].

The mother reported that her daughter had been fine, playing in the yard all morning but in the afternoon, she complained of headaches and stomach pain. She rushed her to the hospital because of the rumors of poison attacks in Jenin. Dr. Hefez thought she may have had some type of infection but her exam was unremarkable. While examining the girl, Hefez was interrupted by the tumultuous arrival of a group of people with another patient. "The new patient was an 18-year-old girl who was quite excited and tried to throw herself off the stretcher while those escorting her tried to restrain her. As with the previous patient, the oxygen mask and intramuscular injection were used instantly. The shouting girl, the excited crowd, the first patient, and her helpless mother together created an atmosphere of utter confusion" [3, p 836]. Dr. Hefez convinced the staff to place the agitated girl in a separate room where she could be examined away from the crowd. Once in a quiet setting, the girl cooperated and Hefez was able to complete his exam. He found no neurologic abnormalities. The girl was able to walk a short distance even though she claimed to be paralyzed. Despite his effort to convince the attending doctors of the importance of keeping her in a separate room, Hefez later found her in a room with three other girls – all who reported the same symptoms.

On the evening of March 27, 64 more young adults living in an eastern neighborhood of Jenin were admitted to hospital with similar symptoms to the other "attacks," this time after seeing or hearing reports of thick smoke pouring out of a speeding car. An article published in the morning paper, *Ha'Aretz* on March 28, stated that preliminary laboratory results confirmed that the Jenin students had been poisoned by nerve gas [3]. There was speculation that the poison had been placed on the classroom curtains, but no evidence was provided. They reported that the Israeli army suspected that someone was trying to provoke the Palestinian population in anticipation of the upcoming protest against Israeli occupation. Palestinian extremists had tried to incite violence in the past. Prominent citizens from Arrabah and Jenin appealed to the United Nations Secretary-General for help. A third and final wave of 'attacks' was the largest, affecting people in the districts of Tolkarem and Hebron and centered around the girls' school in Yattah. Symptoms similar to the prior episodes spread quickly, with 90% of students developing symptoms within 2 hours. Four Israeli soldiers in the area even fell ill. The outbreaks would become known as the Arjenyattah Epidemic for the names of the nearby communities of Arrabah, Jenin, and Yattah [2].

As to who was responsible for the 'poisonings,' it depended on one's political affiliation. The Israelis offered the provocation hypothesis, asserting that a reporter for the Palestinian newspaper *Al'fajr* tried to induce the students to simulate attacks, and noted that no new cases occurred during an imposed curfew [3]. A Palestinian hypothesis was that the Israelis were using chemical weapons to exterminate the Palestinians. Palestinian doctors suggested that the gas was intended to sterilize the affected girls and quoted reports of large amounts of protein in their urine indicating that the ovaries may have been damaged. On April 4, the schools were closed and the epidemic quickly subsided. The Israeli government asked the eminent epidemiologist Baruch Modan to perform a detailed investigation of the episode and after an exhaustive search for physical, chemical and biological factors proved negative, he and his team concluded that it was "mass phenomenon" – a less emotionally charged codeword for mass hysteria. They concluded that the original Arrabah school phase was triggered by an unpleasant odor, hydrogen sulfide, coming from a latrine located in the southeast corner of the schoolyard. Girls in classrooms nearer the latrine had a much higher rate of symptoms than girls in classrooms further away. During recess, rumors spread by friends of the affected girls which led to a "highly contagious process" with many additional cases. Media reports and local rumors set off the second phase in Jenin and neighboring villages, with one major event in particular: the passing car with a faulty exhaust pipe. They found that the third phase was largely triggered by rumors, the media and "local pressure."

Social and political factors played a critical role in propagating the West Bank epidemic. That the suspected cause, a mysterious poison, was believed reflected the sociopolitical fears in the community. It was easy for Palestinian physicians and community leaders to believe this was an attack by the Israelis. This attitude, particularly by the physicians, no doubt acted to reinforce the victims' beliefs, further perpetuating the symptoms. On the other hand, the Israeli press had their own social and political bias, and by expressing their views and opinions, threw "fuel on the fire." Not surprisingly, in this political atmosphere, the Palestinians were not about to accept the Israeli report on the cause of the epidemic and demanded an independent investigation by a politically neutral group of medical experts. The Palestinians agreed to a team of researchers from the US Center for Disease Control (CDC) and the National Institute for Occupational Safety and Health (NIOSH) lead by doctors Philip Landrigan and Bess Miller [4]. After an extensive inquiry that included soil, water and air samples – all of which were negative, they agreed with the Israeli findings that the epidemic was caused by fear and mass suggestion.

Another scare involving the deliberate poisoning of Islamic schoolgirls by Israelis happened in April 1993, after a teenage girl in a village north of Cairo, fainted while reading in front of her class. The incident triggered several of her classmates to follow suit. Media reports about the incident triggered a wave of fainting spells in a number of towns and cities across the country over the next several days and prompting the Egyptian government to declare an emergency. At least 1500 girls between the ages of 9 and 16 were affected by the spells and accompanying nausea, which resulted in the closure of 32 schools. In one incident at a train station in Damanhour, a rumor spread that one of the fainting girls had died. In response, 150 more girls fainted. During the panic, a prominent rumor held that those affected were being deliberately targeted in an Israeli plot to render them sterile [5].

Tainted Chewing Gum Panics

Another scare broke out in Egypt during July 1996, amid rumors of student orgies at a university in the northern city of Mansura. The scare was driven by Member of Parliament, Fathi Mansour, who asserted that Israel had sent agents into the country to sell tainted gum that would heighten the sex drive of young Muslim girls. He claimed to know of at least 15 cases where women had attacked males after chewing the gum [6]. The situation was made worse by the confessions of several girls who told journalists that they had recently engaged in sexual activity after chewing gum. Soon mosques were broadcasting warnings about gum chewing. One student said they were skeptical of the claims but then "we began to hear rumors that a girl had sex with seven boys on campus and another had sex with several men in a car" [7].

No evidence of tainted gum was found. Egyptian tabloids fueled anxieties such as the daily *al Ahrar* which claimed that the gum was designed by a Russian chemist for the Israeli secret service for the purpose of rendering the chewer sterile after three uses, pointing the finger of blame on the Israeli secret service. "The point of this Israeli plan is to reduce the number of births in Arab countries to balance the demographic situation in the area," it claimed. Mansour echoed the claim, "our youth are our hope for the future" [8]. *Washington Post* reporter John Lancaster noted that blaming Israel for various problems facing the country, was something of a national Egyptian pastime. He wrote that recent newspaper stories had linked Israel to the spread of pornography, drug addiction, "sexual promiscuity, AIDS, counterfeit money, health hazards from hormone-laced fruit and, earlier this year, radiation from Israel's Dimona nuclear reactor" [8].

Another gum scare took place in 1997, amid rumors that strawberry-flavored gum had been laced with sex hormones that were said to make them 'crazy for sex,' but would eventually render them sterile. Once again it was said to have been an Israeli plot. *The Times of Israel* only made the situation worse by claiming that 200 tons of aphrodisiac gum had recently been confiscated by Palestinian forces and that the gum was being sold by Israeli agents "so that Palestinian women will become prostitutes and be easily recruited as spies" [9]. In 2009, a third chewing gum scare broke out with claims by pro-Palestinian group Hamas that Israel was slipping aphrodisiac chewing gum to Palestinian girls and boys. The latest panic was reportedly touched off when a father witnessed his daughter acting oddly after chewing on gum. One journalist offered an alternative explanation for the girl's actions: puberty [10].

Other Pseudo-Poisonings

On the night of April 9, 1989, during a period of political upheaval in the former Soviet state of Georgia, an estimated 10,000 people attended an anti-Soviet rally in the capital of Tbilisi. During the event, Soviet troops dispersed the gathering by spraying tear gas and other chemical irritants. As a result, about 4000 participants sought medical assistance at nearby hospitals, of which 543 patients were admitted. At least 20 deaths were recorded. While two of the chemicals used were identified, the nature of a mysterious third agent, remained a mystery until an investigation by Dr. Barry Rumack, of the University of Colorado Medical Center who visited the country shortly after the attack. After analyzing the contents of a cannister found at the scene, he was able to determine the third substance was chloropicrin – a powerful insecticide that was used as a chemical weapon during the First World War and can affect the lungs, eyes, skin, nose and throat [11].

Near the end of a 40-day period of national mourning for the dead, a group of visiting American physicians were meeting with local health officials over the incident when they were suddenly interrupted – about 400 children from nearby schools had just been rushed to several hospitals with symptoms nearly identical to those who had been at the rally. Symptoms included skins rash, burning eyes, dry throats, and abdominal pain. Nearly all of the patients were adolescent girls. Psychiatrist Ruth Baron of the Harvard Medical School was able to examine some of the affected students. She and a group of French medical practitioners examined some 40 patients at a local pediatric hospital and concluded that the girls were suffering from mass hysteria. She believed that the most likely precipitating cause "was the fact that the forty-day Georgian mourning period for the dead demonstrators was about to end, protests would be allowed again, many of those hospitalized had siblings or friends injured on April 9, and it was all too much to bear" [11, p 604]. In an attempt to soothe the nerves of jittery parents, and not appear insensitive to the girls' plight, they announced that the students were exhibiting "catastrophic reaction syndrome" and they would recover soon.

In December 2005, reports emerged of mass poisonings at schools in the Shelkovsk region of the Russian Republic of Chechnya, which was attributed to Russian agents. Symptoms included convulsions, seizures, fainting spells, headaches, difficulty breathing and numbness. The complaints spread quickly to schools in nearby villages. Eventually, nearly 100 adolescent girls were stricken. When Russian government health personnel investigated the outbreak and announced their diagnosis of mass psychogenic illness, it was met with vehement opposition from local residents and members of the medical community. One of the physicians who treated the first cases and diagnosed them with "an intoxication of unknown aetiology," Vaha Ehselayev, was incredulous at this assessment, believing it to have been a government coverup. "I believe that there is a poisonous agent in the victims' schools. But the political situation is such that it has to be denied. We don't know what the agent was. We don't have the resources to find out," he said [12]. However, the commission tasked with investigating the outbreak, organized by government officials in Moscow and Grozny, said it could find no evidence that the students were poisoned, that the school grounds were found to have been safe, leading "to the conclusion that there was an outbreak of mass hysteria in the Shelkovsk region related to the prolonged emergency situation in the Chechen Republic" [12].

In the wake of strong opposition to the diagnosis of mass hysteria by parents and health professionals in Chechnya, symptoms in many of the victims lingered for months. That was when Chechen psychologist, Khapta Akhmedova, convinced that the diagnosis of mass hysteria was correct, began to set up a program aimed at reassuring victims that stress was the underlying cause. By October 2006, they had all been released from the hospital and most had returned to school [13]. British journalist Laura Spinney who researched the episode, noted the crucial role that belief played in the recovery, and the importance of positive reassurance. "In Shelkovsk, teachers, parents and doctors continue to reject the Russian verdict of mass hysteria, even though psychological treatment is the only thing that has helped their children. What will it take to cure those who remain sick? Perhaps an acknowledgement from those around them that the only thing poisoning them is their own anxiety" [13]. It is significant that the 'poisonings' took place amid longstanding political discord between Russia and Chechnya which became pronounced in the early 1990s and the breakup of the former

Soviet Union. Ever since this time, separatists have waged an ideological campaign to create an independent Islamic state; a campaign that has demonized the Russian government and sown distrust of the Kremlin.

Kosovo

In March 1990, alarming news reports began to circulate about the mass poisoning of thousands of young people in the Serbian province of Kosovo. At the time, the region was a hotbed of ethnic tensions between Serbs and Albanians. Divisions between the two rival groups were so deep that classes in elementary and high schools were even segregated along ethnic lines [14]. The first casualties were reported on March 14, then quickly spread. By March 23, it was being reported that 417 people, mostly students from the small city of Besiana, were receiving medical attention for what appeared to be poisoning. Over the next few days, hundreds of more people were stricken. Authorities also noted an oddity: virtually all of those affected with headaches, dizziness, sore throats, fainting spells, and vomiting, were ethnic Albanians. Other symptoms included chest pain, cramps, burning sensations, over-breathing, and dry mouth [15]. In the ensuing days and weeks, many news reports suggested the possibility that a neurotoxin was used. The tenor of some of these stories was critical of Yugoslav authorities. For instance, soon after the episode began, the largest newspaper in the Albanian capital of Tirana, published a commentary blaming Yugoslav authorities for orchestrating the 'poisoning.' It stated in part: "It seems like the firearms used against the Kosovo people since 1981, has not been effective enough. Therefore, a new more effective weapon has been invented, more psychologically directed: a poisoning... Serbs were those who demanded segregation in the schools and dormitories... poisonings such as the Yugoslav type have not been heard of even in South African ghettos" [14]. By mid-April, over 4000 Albanians had been stricken.

Three separate sets of researchers have published their analysis of the episode – each concluding that it was caused by mass psychogenic illness [16–18]. Among them was Kuwaiti epidemiologist Dr. Zoran Radovanovic who would publish his findings in the *European Journal of Epidemiology*. In the wake of negative tests for toxins or an organic cause, he noted some key signs of mass hysteria: rapid onset and recovery in most victims who were overwhelmingly teenage girls exhibiting the symptoms of anxiety such as hyperventilation. There was one particularly telling sign of the psychogenic nature of the outbreak: the pattern of spread as only one ethnic group was stricken. Radovanovic writes: "Not a single non-Albanian student or adult was affected. This feature of the epidemic appears to be the most indisputable one, since neither a doctor, nor a layman, including journalists in search for exceptions, ever challenged it" [15, p 110]. He traced the outbreak to a confluence of events: the presence of poisoning rumors, ethnic tension, suspicion and mistrust, the presence of unfamiliar odors and substances, and media stories that fanned poisoning suspicions. A coincidental spike in the number of respiratory infections during the period further stoked anxieties [15, p 111]. Early in the outbreak, a rumor spread within the Albanian community that the Serbs had sprayed an unknown chemical into the classrooms of the affected students. Generating further hostility and anger, some Serbian government officials accused those complaining of symptoms of faking [15, p 101]. Pre-existing tensions were so great that during the previous year when a polio vaccine was being administered among Albanians, a panic ensued after rumors that it was being used to secretly sterilize their children. Many ran away from the vaccination sites; some leaping out of windows as high as two stories! [15, p 107].

In September and October of 1997, the appearance of headaches, breathing problems, stomach cramps, and anxiety attacks affected about 1000 ethnic Albanian students in the Macedonian town of Tetovo, about 140 km south of Kosovo. Amid continuing ethnic strife, those who were unwell blamed their neighbors for poisoning them. A subsequent investigation by the World Health Organization ruled out an infectious agent or toxin. The head of the investigation team, Zsuzsanna Jakab, said that a foul odor was noticed just prior to the panic, after which a few real cases of food poisoning or influenza laid the foundation for the mass suggestion that was to follow [19, 20]. The episode occurred amidst a backdrop of longstanding Albanian-Macedonian ethnic conflict [21]. As with the events in Kosovo during 1990, a similar pattern emerged as the WHO found that "the disease only affected ethnic Albanian students in certain schools." A more short-term response to fears of an attack by a hostile foreign actor took place during the Persian Gulf War. At the time, there were grave fears in Israel that Saddam Hussein would fire Scud missiles containing poison gas at Israel. While the missiles were eventually fired, they contained no chemical warheads. In spite of this, after the first attack, about 40% of civilians in the immediate vicinity exhibited breathing problems [22].

Afghanistan

Over the past decade, there have been dozens of reported attacks involving the mass poisoning of Afghan schoolgirls perpetrated by the Taliban government in exile which controls parts of the war-torn country. For instance, in May 2018, the Chinese Xinhua News Agency reported that "45 Afghan girl students were poisoned following a suspected gas attack in the northern province of Takhar on Thursday, local police said" [23]. These poisoning reports began as early as 2009, the same year that the *Stateman* published the headline: "Afghan Schoolgirls Targeted in 'Taliban Gas Attack'" [24]. The following year, *The International Herald Tribune* proclaimed: "Poison Gas Sickened Afghan Girls." [25]. In 2015, the *New York Daily News* carried the story: "More than 100 Afghan Schoolgirls, Teachers Poisoned in Suspected Taliban Attack" [26]. In 2017, CNN's Jason Hanna asserted matter-of-factly that "Numerous schoolgirls have been attacked in Afghanistan over the past two decades, in part to dissuade them and others from attending school…Hundreds have been hospitalized over the years, for example, because of poisoning attacks at their schools…" [27]. But take a closer look at these accounts and you will notice something odd: not a single schoolgirl has died or been seriously harmed. After each incident, those who were taken to local hospitals quickly recovered and were released. Symptoms included headaches, dizziness, fainting, nausea, vomiting, and general weakness.

This unusual pattern was recognized in 2012 when The World Health Organization (WHO) released the results of a study on 'attacks taking place between 2009 and 2012. Investigators looked at incidents in 22 schools involving 1634 patients over the period and concluded that in every instance, the cause was "mass psychogenic illness." While many Afghans have blamed the Taliban forces who are vehemently opposed to girls attending school, Taliban spokesmen have always denied their involvement. Most episodes were triggered by an unfamiliar odor that was attributed to a chemical or biological terror attack, although in some cases it was rumors of a poisoned water supply [28]. While the WHO has published a one-page summary of their findings, the full report has never been released. A WHO representative familiar with the study says that based on blood, urine and water samples, there was "No conclusive evidence of deliberate poisoning." In 2013, Afghan journalist Matthieu Aikins uncovered the existence of two other studies into the 'mass poisonings' – conducted by The North Atlantic Treaty Organization (NATO), and the United Nations. Both reached the same conclusion as the WHO study: the schoolgirl 'poisonings' were mass hysteria [29].

A search of ProQuest Newsstand which includes the text of over 1300 newspapers, news websites, and blogs from around the world, failed to identify a single confirmed case a mass poisoning at an Afghan school [30]. The first known incident occurred in Khost province in 2004 after three girls reportedly fell sick [31, 32]. A Taliban spokesman denied any responsibility [33]. On many occasions since, Taliban officials have continued to vehemently deny any involvement [34], and emphasized that such actions were unIslamic and in violation of Sharia law [35]. An alarming aspect to these 'attacks' is that over the past decade, many innocent people have been arrested and charged with the 'poisonings,' and Afghan newspapers have called for harsh penalties for the perpetrators [36]. In July 2012, Afghanistan's national security agency released videotaped confessions of several suspects including two 17-year-old students [37]. In response, the United Nations Human Rights Unit protested their validity [29, 38]. Between August and September 2015, several mass poisoning incidents at girls' schools were reported in Herat Province involving poisoned air or water. The incidents were confined to the Provincial capital city of Herat [39–43]. Three separate investigations of the Herat 'attacks' by the Afghan Ministry of Education and the International Assistance Mission (IAM), concluded that psychogenic illness was the cause [44–46].

References

1. Merton R. The self-fulfilling prophecy. Antioch Rev. 1948;8:193–210. See p. 195.
2. Modan B, Tirosh M, Weissenberg E, Acker C, Swartz T, Costin C, et al. The Arjenyattah epidemic. Lancet. 1983;2:1472–4.
3. Hefez A. The role of the press and the medical community in an epidemic of mysterious gas poisoning in the Jordan West Bank. Am J Psych. 1985;142:833–7.

4. Landrigan PJ, Miller B. The Arjenyattah epidemic: home interview data and toxicological aspects. Lancet. 1983;2:1474–6.
5. Spring fever. The Fortean Times (London). 1993;69:16.
6. La Guardia A. The belly-dancer and the envoy. The Spectator (London). 1997;279(8830):28–9.
7. Jehl D. Of college girls betrayed and vile chewing gum. The New York Times. 10 July 1996.
8. Lancaster J. Sabotaging Egypt, by gum: Cairo tabloids claim Israel snuck aphrodisiacs into the chaw. The Washington Post. 10 July 1996;Sect. A:12.
9. Bartholomew RE, Rickard B. Mass hysteria in schools: a worldwide history since 1566. Jefferson: McFarland; 2014. p. 60.
10. Next, the Gaza Strip? The New York Daily News. 15 July 2009, p. 28.
11. Goldsmith M. Physicians with Georgia on their minds. JAMA. 1989;262:603–4.
12. Politkovskaya A. Poison in the air… The Guardian. 1 Mar 2006. p. 12.
13. Spinney L. Terror's hidden ally. New Scientist. 2006;192(2573):24.
14. Luci N, Markovic P. Events and sites of difference: marking self and other in Kosova. In: Kolstø P, editor. Media discourse and the Yugoslav conflicts: representations of self and other. New York: Routledge; 2009. p. 83–104. See p. 91.
15. Radovanovic Z. On the origin of mass casualty incidents in Kosovo, Yugoslavia, in 1990. Eur J Epidemiol. 1996;12:101–13.
16. Federal Commission of Experts. Report of mass outbreak of health disorders in Kosovo. Beograd: Federal Ministry of Labour, Health, Veteran Affairs and Social Policy; 1990.
17. Hay A, Foran J. Yugoslavia: poisoning or epidemic hysteria in Kosovo? Lancet. 1991;338:1196.
18. Radovanovic Z. Health concerns in Kosova. BMJ. 1994;308(6921):138.
19. MacKenzie D. Ethnic strife triggers psychosomatic illness. New Scientist. 1997;153(2066):5.
20. Mass Hysteria: Telling the truth to the terrified. The Economist. 18 May 2006.
21. Demjaha A. The State of inter-ethnic relations in Macedonia after 16 years of the Ohrid agreement. SEEU Review. 2017;2(2):8–31.
22. Carmeli A, Liberman N, Mevorach L. Anxiety-related somatic reactions during missile attacks. Isr J Med Sci. 1991;27:677–80.
23. 45 School girls hospitalized in suspected gas attack in N. Afghanistan, Xinhua News Agency. 3 May 2018.
24. Afghan schoolgirls targeted in 'Taliban gas attacks.' The Statesman (New Delhi, India). 15 May 2009.
25. Nordland R. Poison gas sickened Afghan schoolgirls. The International Herald Tribune (Paris). 1 Sept 2010. p. 8.
26. Wagner M. More Than 100 Afghan schoolgirls, teachers, poisoned in suspected Taliban attack. The New York Daily News. 31 Aug 2015.
27. Hanna J. Other times terror attacks targeted children. CNN (Atlanta, GA). 23 May 2017.
28. Mass psychogenic illness in Afghanistan. WHO Weekly Epidemiological Monitor. 27 May 2012;5.
29. Aikins M. The 'poisoned' schoolgirls of Afghanistan. The New York Times. 25 Apr 2013.
30. The sources include numerous papers of record such as The New York Times, The Chicago Tribune, Los Angeles Times, The Guardian, The Wall Street Journal, The Washington Post, USA Today, and the The Boston Globe.
31. Schoolgirls poisoned. The Journal (Newcastle-upon-Tyne, UK). 3 May 2004. p. 6.
32. Bearup G. Girls 'poisoned' by militants for going to school. The Guardian. 3 May 2004.
33. Neo-Taliban denies poisoning girls, Afghan report. Radio Free Europe Radio Liberty. 13 May 2004. https://www.rferl.org/a/1340574.html. Accessed 15 Oct 2019.
34. 'Poison' panic in girls' schools. Killid Weekly (Kabul). 11 June 2012.
35. Taliban deny poison attacks on girls' schools. BBC News. 27 May 2012.
36. More Takhar school girls poisoned as suspects arrested. Tolo News (Kabul). 5 June 2012.
37. Aikins M. Toxic panic: the Taliban are accused of poisoning more than 1,000 Afghan schoolgirls. But did they? Examining the evidence. Newsweek (Pacific edition). 16 July 2012.

38. Hodge N, Totakhil H. World News: Afghan torture allegations rattle relations with U.N. Wall Street Journal. 12 July 2012;Sect. A:13.
39. Variyar M. Afghanistan: Gas poisoning lands over 100 schoolgirls in hospital in Herat. International Business Times. 13 Aug 2015.
40. Hundreds of Afghan schoolgirls in hospital after suspected poison gas attacks. Anadolu Agency (Ankara, Turkey). 3 Sept 2015.
41. Bruton FB, Rahim F. School poisoning? Dozens of girls fall ill in Herat, Afghanistan. NBC News. 31 Aug 2015. https://www.nbcnews.com/news/world/school-poisoning-dozens-girls-fall-ill-herat-afghanistan-n418616. Accessed 1 Nov 2019.
42. Schoolgirls, teachers poisoned in Herat: officials, 2015. TOLO News (Kabul, Afghanistan). 5 Sept 2015.
43. Najm AF, Lockery S. Timeline of the events at Herat. Internal International Assistance Mission report. 2015.
44. Niayzi A, Sadequ S, Joya S, Faizi S, Rasoli A, Moaid K, et al. Report on case control study poisoning in Herat school students. Ministry of Education, Afghanistan, Final Report. 24 Nov 2015, 3pp.
45. Najm AF. Assessment report...of poisoning of school students in Herat province. Community Health Project, International Assistance Mission (Afghanistan); 2015, 4pp.
46. Bartholomew RE, Lockery S, Najm AF. Terror attacks that never were: myths of poison gas attacks in history and more recently on Afghan schoolgirls. The Skeptic (Altadena, CA). 2016;21(3):44–9.

The Social Construction of 'Havana Syndrome'

11

A wise man, therefore, proportions his belief to the evidence.

–David Hume [1]

Many years ago, an American zoologist told of visiting a tribe in a remote part of Africa. Suddenly, clouds of billowing dust appeared in the distance and began slowly moving towards him. An elder tribesman began shouting excitedly, 'Look! Giant dragonflies! Giant dragonflies!' As the cloud grew closer, an outline of stampeding elephants began to take shape. The zoologist turned to the man and said, 'Those aren't dragonflies, they're elephants!' to which the man proclaimed: 'Look! The giant dragonflies have turned into elephants!' [2]. Human beings have a remarkable capacity for self-deception. Throughout history, people have come to believe in the existence of an array of imaginary assailants, from witches and demons to mad gassers and poisoning plots by foreign agents – beliefs that made people sick based solely on the power of suggestion. The events in Cuba are just the latest in a long list of scares involving phantom attackers who stepped out of the shadows to terrorize small groups and communities. Each of these episodes occurred in an anxiety-filled atmosphere, within a unique social and cultural backdrop that rendered the threat plausible.

Our worldview is central to shaping how we interpret, order, and perceive reality. As Anthropologist John Connor observes, "a forest…will be perceived quite differently by a botanist, an entomologist, a logger, a poet, and a little boy who is lost" [3]. A person's belief system changes how they perceive the world. What then, was the crucial outlook of American Embassy employees just prior to the 'attacks' in Cuba? They were in a hostile foreign country that had a history of harassment against American diplomats – to the point of dumping human feces on living room floors and poisoning pets. They were under relentless surveillance and could not even relax in their own homes as agents frequently entered their residences while they were asleep or away. When the first few diplomats began to hear strange noises, they were unsure of what to make of them, but a belief soon emerged that they were being harassed. Put another way, instead of thinking horses, their worldview predisposed them to

© Springer Nature Switzerland AG 2020
R. W. Baloh, R. E. Bartholomew, *Havana Syndrome*,
https://doi.org/10.1007/978-3-030-40746-9_11

assume that they were hearing the hoofbeats of zebras. However, when State Department officials accepted the more exotic hypothesis and assumed that they were the victims of sonic attacks, they left the realm of speculation and the possible and entered the world of science fiction and unicorns. Recordings made by some of the victims were examined by experts in acoustical physics and entomology, concluding that they were the mating calls of crickets and cicadas [4–5]. When a third of the Embassy patients studied reported that these and similar sounds had damaged their hearing, this bred confusion because these insects cannot generate sounds loud enough to cause hearing loss. But when Dr. Michael Hoffer and his team published the results of their hearing tests, while many patients *thought* they had suffered hearing loss, only two had, both of whom had hearing problems *before* going to Cuba [6].

Sonic Weapons and Science Fiction

Throughout this saga, our institutions have failed us. The American Government was too quick to jump to conclusions that are not commensurate with the facts and have refused to admit they may have been wrong. They have steadfastly refused to release Freedom of Information documents. At times major media outlets known for their high journalist standards such as 60 *Minutes* and *The New Yorker*, have engaged in shoddy reporting, releasing sensational, one-sided stories while leaving out voices of dissent. Even our scientific institutions like the *Journal of the American Medical Association* have failed to meet the normal standard of scientific research, sowing confusion and eroding confidence in the science. But these are temporary aberrations. The government, the media, and our scientific institutions are strong and self-policing; they eventually right themselves. Embassy workers have contradicted dubious claims by scientists and journalists that some of the American diplomats at the Cuban Embassy were unaware that their colleagues had fallen ill. Many media outlets have published the views of dissenting scientists. Even the *Journal of the American Medical Association*, which had done so much to promote the scare by publishing not one but two poorly conceived studies, did publish a host of opposing views by scientists who attacked their conclusions. Several journals have taken up the cause, harshly criticizing the dubious studies claiming a link between 'Havana Syndrome' and brain damage and hearing loss in such publications as the *Journal of the Royal Society of Medicine*, *The International Journal of Social Psychiatry*, *The Swiss Medical Weekly*, *Scientific American*, *Cortex*, and others.

Had State Department officials done their homework, they would have realized that a Buck Rogers-style sonic weapon that could penetrate the walls of houses and hotels and zap their target, would violate the laws of physics. Sound waves dissipate rapidly with distance; most of the energy would bounce harmlessly off the walls before finding their target. Any ultrasound-generating devices in a room would be obvious to anyone inside. While ultrasound can potentially damage hearing, aside from the two diplomats with pre-existing hearing problems, none of the others tested had hearing loss. There is also no compelling evidence that it can cause brain trauma. Claims of a microwave attack are equally far-fetched. In order to damage the brain, the energy required would be so intense that it would burn the victim! While most embassy staff and their families who became ill reported hearing a sound that was associated with the onset of their symptoms, the notion that audible sound can damage the brain is implausible. Profound hearing loss would occur long before there was any effect on the brain. Furthermore, the short duration of the sound exposure reported by most subjects and the fact that several did not even hear it, effectively rules out audible sound as a cause of their symptoms. An infrasound device that could produce enough energy to damage the brain would have to be large and would likely pose as much danger to the operators as the targets. It is difficult to focus infrasound waves and clearly, anyone in the vicinity would feel the vibration – something that did not happen in Cuba as on several occasions, people in the same room as the victim, heard and felt nothing. High-frequency ultrasound waves are easier to focus and very high frequency ultrasound in the range of 20,000 Hertz have been used to break up kidney stones. Yet, while the US Government experimented with ultrasound ray guns in the 1990s, it gave up because the waves do not travel long distances, the energy dissipates too rapidly, and they are easily impeded.

While three studies have lent credence to claims that a mysterious energy force harmed the diplomats in Cuba – be it sonic, microwave or otherwise, none were supported by the evidence, and each study contained significant errors. The research teams in Miami and Pennsylvania were chosen by the government and given exclusive access to their patients. This may have influenced their interpretation of the data; seeing what they wanted to see in order to unconsciously please those who had entrusted them with their patients. How else can you explain their drawing conclusions that were not warranted by the evidence? A similar confirmation bias may be at work in the Canadian fumigation study by overlooking the different experiences of the American and Canadian diplomats, and the conspicuous absence of non-diplomats who worked at the embassies.

This entire affair has been muddled by the media reporting speculation by experts in various fields, that has no underpinning in fact. A classic example was the reporting by CBS News in September 2018, surrounding a briefing of the Joint Chiefs of Staff on possible causes of the 'attacks' in Cuba by James Giordano, Chief of Neuroethics Studies at Georgetown University. He told them that the most likely cause was "some form of electromagnetic pulse generation and/or hypersonic generation that would then utilize the architecture of the skull to create something of an energetic amplifier or lens to induce a cavitational effect that would then induce the type of pathologic changes that would then induce the constellation of signs and symptoms that we're seeing in these patients." While Giordano's explanation may sound erudite and scientific, it was pure speculation and lacking in any concrete supporting evidence, but that did not stop CBS and other media outlets from reporting on it and giving it an air of credibility as no skeptics were quoted to counter his claim [7].

A Pattern Emerges

State Department officials and physicians examining the data on the Havana patients have made a curious observation, the significance of which cannot be overstated. During a press briefing in Washington DC on September 28, 2017, spokeswoman

Heather Nauert observed: "We have never seen this anyplace in the world before" [8]. Doctors treating the patients have made similar observations, using such terms as "novel clinical entity" [9] and "new syndrome" [10]. In his testimony before the Senate Foreign Relations Committee, State Department doctor Charles Rosenfarb concurred with this assessment, noting that what may be a "novel syndrome" was proving to be a challenge to understand [11]. What might this new syndrome be, and why has it not been identified before now? The answer is – it has.

Over the past 150 years, soldiers returning from combat have been diagnosed with a novel syndrome for which no organic cause could be found. Despite the array of names given to it, the symptoms have remained remarkably uniform. Some of the most common complaints include headaches, dizziness, disorientation, forgetfulness, difficulty concentrating, fatigue, insomnia, chest pain, and impaired sight and hearing. Occasionally, doctors have described their cognitive function as resembling *concussion-like symptoms but without a concussion*. During the Civil War, it was called Da Costa Syndrome after the physician who first recognized it, Jacob Da Costa. In World War I, doctors named it shell shock or Soldier's Heart. Troops fighting in World War II were diagnosed with combat stress reaction and war neurosis. In Vietnam War veterans the term was post-traumatic stress disorder. More recently, vets returning from deployment in the Middle East were diagnosed with Gulf War Syndrome. These psychogenic symptoms associated with American soldiers living under continuous stress are virtually identical to those reported by the US diplomats working under continuous surveillance while living on foreign soil under the specter of the Cold War.

The symptoms of shell shock in World War I and war neurosis during the Second World War, clearly overlap with the symptoms reported by patients who reported "acoustic attacks." Medical personnel in both wars eventually concluded that the best way to manage soldiers with shell shock and war neurosis was to treat them near the front providing reassurance and expectation of a rapid recovery and using simple procedures such as rest, sleep and supportive psychotherapy. *Soldiers who were sent home to specialized clinics often developed chronic symptoms related to the specialty of the referred clinic and rarely returned to the military* whereas the great majority of those treated near the front recovered within a few weeks. There are obvious parallels between post-traumatic stress disorder (PTSD) and the embassy syndrome. Symptoms began after a stressful event, an "acoustic attack" in a foreign country, and complaints including anxiety and depression, typically become chronic. Some of the embassy staff and families met the diagnostic criteria for PTSD. There is also a clear overlap between PTSD and mild traumatic brain injury. The concept of a brain injury that is bad enough to cause symptoms but without obvious neurological findings has become popular as soldiers from the Afghanistan and Iraq wars have returned home complaining of a range of chronic symptoms including memory and cognitive deficits such as difficulty with decision-making. Some of these soldiers were exposed to blasts but most were not anywhere near a blast when the symptoms began. The overlap in symptoms of 'Havana Syndrome' with those of mild traumatic brain injury was the reason the embassy patients were referred to a traumatic brain injury clinic in the first place. But what is the evidence that the soldiers or the embassy victims had a brain injury? Standard neurological examinations and magnetic resonance imaging (MRI) of the brain have been consistently normal. Abnormalities on neuropsychological, balance, and eye movement testing are nonspecific indicating brain malfunctioning but not brain injury and these abnormalities are commonly seen in patients with a wide range of psychogenic illnesses. It has been suggested that newer, more specialized brain imaging techniques may be able to identify subtle changes in the brain in people with mild traumatic brain injury but minor abnormalities are common. Telling a person that they have a brain injury has obvious implications for their long-term expectations. It is well known that negative expectations often lead to negative outcomes: the nocebo effect [12].

Chronic symptoms that persist beyond 3 months after a head trauma are better predicted by pre-concussion psychosocial factors than by acute symptoms or the nature of the head injury [13]. To suggest that someone has a brain injury because they have symptoms that overlap with post-concussion symptoms is illogical. Finally, there are similarities between the Gulf War Syndrome and 'Havana Syndrome.' Both groups had a wide range of overlapping symptoms including cognitive and chronic mood disorders. Unlike the soldiers in Afghanistan and Iraq, relatively few of the Gulf War soldiers were exposed to blast injuries. Gulf War Syndrome victims spent months in the desert housed in barracks hearing rumors of potential chemical and biological weapons and dangerous side effects from vaccines and medications they had received. 'Havana Syndrome' victims spent months in a potentially hostile country hearing rumors of mysterious sonic weapons that could injure their brains. As with the embassy victims, Gulf War victims underwent extensive investigations looking for environmental toxins and other exposures that might have caused the symptoms, but none were found.

Historical Parallels

The evidence that US Embassy personnel in Cuba were the victims of mass psychogenic illness, also known as mass hysteria, is overwhelming. The symptoms in Cuba closely parallel several recent illness clusters that have been identified as outbreaks of mass psychogenic illness, after having been initially diagnosed as an attack with chemical weapons by a hostile foreign government. Despite media speculation fueling anxiety and initial controversy surrounding these diagnoses, there is a consensus within the medical community that they were psychogenic in nature. In 1983, in the Israeli occupied West Bank, the outbreak was confined to a single ethnic group that believed they were being targeted with poison gas by Israeli agents: Palestinian schoolgirls. In 1990, the 'mass poisoning' of over 4000 residents of Kosovo and was later diagnosed as mass hysteria in no less than 3 separate studies, was confined to ethnic Albanians. During December 2005, in the Russian Republic of Chechnya, it was only Chechnyan students who were stricken. The tendency for mass hysteria to affect specific groups is telling, for chemical and biological agents cannot discriminate along ethnic lines, especially in the diffuse communitywide outbreaks just cited. This same pattern held true in Cuba: only diplomatic staff or their families were affected and later diagnosed with "medically confirmed symptoms." The Canadian diplomats who were reportedly affected were also Embassy staff or their families, who reported their symptoms only after being alerted by US officials. While an attack by a foreign government using sound may appear unique, as we have seen in Chaps. 6 and 7, there is a considerable literature dating back centuries involving claims of sound waves causing ill-health. Scientists have carefully examined these assertions and a clear consensus has emerged: they were the result of mass psychogenic illness and the Nocebo Effect. Benjamin Franklin's glass armonica is a classic example. When it was first invented, it was widely touted as being beneficial to health. There were many instances of people who were listening to the armonica who suddenly felt better. However, by the early nineteenth century and rumors that the device was injurious to health, the exact opposite happened, and people began attributing their illnesses to the armonica. This changing perception was clearly psychological and driven by expectation.

Claims of 'telephone tinnitus' and 'acoustical shock' by telephone operators dating back to the late nineteenth century are just two more examples of sound purported to have caused illness in response to the appearance of new technologies. There is now a consensus that both conditions were psychogenic. In the case of 'acoustical shock,' some scientists observed that the victims were suffering from *concussion-like symptoms*. Reports of 'The Hum' in many parts of the world have been blamed for an array of psychogenic symptoms starting in about 1980, coinciding with a flurry of alarming media stories on the phenomenon. Conspicuously, reports of similar sounds prior to this time only elicited annoyance and insomnia. There are many similarities between the sounds reported by hummers and 'Havana Syndrome.' The sounds were typically very localized so that if the person went outside or left the room where the sound was heard, it disappeared. Some people in both groups reported feeling either pressure or vibration that seemed to come from the same direction as the sound. There were examples where one individual in the room heard the sound while another in the same room heard nothing. People made recordings of the sound, yet the source could not be pinpointed. The descriptions and recordings of the sounds varied greatly in both groups suggesting that there were multiple sound sources. One apparent difference between the two groups was the frequency of the sound they reported. Most hummers reported low frequency sounds whereas the embassy personnel usually described higher frequency sounds although a few described the sound as a hum and it is common for people to confuse frequency and loudness. And of course, people living near wind turbines have complained that the sound of the turning blades makes them sick, yet many common, ever-present sounds such as human respiration produces higher levels of sub-audible sound. The social patterning of Wind Turbine Syndrome is evident. For instance, nearly three-quarters of all complaints in Australia come from just six farms that were the focus of negative media publicity after being targeted by wind farm opponents. This mysterious 'new syndrome' is driven by the expectation of ill health through the Nocebo Effect where people can literally think themselves to feel sick.

The events in Cuba also parallel the literature on mass hysteria and social delusions involving phantom assailants. In some cases, these 'attackers' were believed to have sprayed poison gas to make people sick. Studies of the 'mad gasser' of Virginia during the 1930s and the Illinois 'gasser' of 1944, were both sparked by an initial sensational case that received dramatic news coverage about 'gassings' that made the existence of these imaginary assailants appear real. During this period, many conferences on international disarmament were held and attempts were made to ban all chemical weapons. The American preoccupation with this issue provided the backdrop to the 1938 'War of the Worlds' Martian invasion scare in the United States. Psychologist Hadley Cantril found that 20% of listeners interviewed who thought the 'attacks' were real, believed that the announcer was mistaken and that the 'Martian attack' was a poison gas raid, not by extraterrestrials, but the German military. As one respondent observed: "The announcer said a meteor had fallen from Mars and I was sure that he thought that, but in the back of my head I had the idea that the meteor was just a camouflage…and the Germans were attacking us with gas bombs [14]." What one historian referred to at this time as "the poison gas scare" even shaped the form of the gasser panics [15]. For instance, in Virginia, the use of chlorine gas was initially suspected by authorities, while in Illinois, it was chloropicrin: both chemicals that were used during World War I and were still in the arsenals of some countries into the 1940s.

Common Misperceptions

While historically most cases of mass psychogenic illness have taken place in schools and factories and mostly affected females, there are reports of outbreaks in all-boy schools. One of the largest episodes on American soil in the twentieth century occurred at a naval training center in San Diego, California during the summer of 1998, amid a backdrop of brush fires and a mysterious odor. In all, 164 males experienced dizziness, breathing difficulties and to a lesser extent, vomiting. Tensions were heightened after some recruits were given mouth-to-mouth resuscitation after several medics who had just arrived on the scene, believed that some young men were dying. This unusual set of circumstances generated extreme anxiety among the remaining recruits. Investigators found that those who witnessed the 'resuscitations' or saw others exhibit symptoms, were three times more likely to report symptoms [16]. And of course, the largest known outbreaks of psychogenic illness in history have predominantly involved males: the variously named combat syndromes beginning with studies of the American Civil War to the Afghan and Iraq War syndromes.

The idea that people with mass psychogenic illness are malingering or faking symptoms has been thoroughly discredited. People with psychogenic illness have real symptoms due to changes in brain and body physiology [12]. Although some physicians have been skeptical of patients with psychogenic illness from the earliest times, there is little evidence for fakery or malingering. If a physician shows even the slightest hint of skepticism towards a patient's symptoms, there is little chance of helping the patient. However, when the medical and legal systems become involved, perverse incentives may prolong symptoms and diminish the chance of recovery.

Finally, the notion that mass psychogenic illnesses are short-lived and do not become chronic simply ignores the numerous examples of mass psychogenic illnesses with chronic symptoms described throughout this book. The epidemics of mass psychogenic illness triggered by the wars of the twentieth century described in Chap. 4 are clear examples of chronic mass psychogenic illness. Shell shock, war neurosis, post-traumatic stress syndrome and the Gulf War Syndrome all produced chronic symptoms. Interestingly, there is strong evidence that early recognition along with supportive therapy and reassurance can decrease the likelihood that symptoms will become chronic. Even in the outbreaks of mass psychogenic illness in schools, communities, and workplaces where symptoms were brief in most, some people developed chronic symptoms. Referrals to specialized clinics increased the risk of developing chronic symptoms.

Mass psychogenic illness and the social panics that often accompany them are significant health and social problems. The associated financial costs can be staggering. One series of outbreaks among Belgian schoolchildren in the summer of 1999, cost the Coca-Cola Company upwards of a quarter of a billion dollars in lost revenues over false concerns about tainted products [17]. In 2007, a group of Australian schoolgirls who fainted while being inoculated for human papillomavirus, is estimated to have wiped AU$1 billion from the stock value of the corporation producing the Gardasil vaccine [18]. Unfounded safety concerns gave momentum to the anti-vaccination lobby which swayed parents to forego vaccinations for their daughters, increasing their susceptibility to cervical cancer [19, 20]. In 1983, odor from a toilet at a girls' school in the Israeli occupied West Bank prompted fears that students had been poisoned by Mossad agents. In response, nearly a thousand Palestinian schoolgirls developed psychogenic symptoms and set into motion a series of events that led to a UN resolution condemning the 'attack' and stoked war fears between Israel and its neighbors. Likewise, claims of an attack on American diplomats in Havana have created an atmosphere of suspicion and distrust between the two countries and threatens to set relations back to the Cold War era. Blaming Russia or other foreign actors such as China for perpetrating the 'attacks' along with the Cubans, have unnecessarily raised diplomatic tensions. State Department warnings about visiting Cuba because of the risk of 'attacks,' has also resulted in a significant drop in tourist revenue [21, 22].

In 1958, author Graham Greene, a former member of the British spy service MI6 in World War II, published the novel *Our Man in Havana*, mocking intelligence agencies and their tendency to give undue weight to local informants with little supporting evidence. Set in Havana during the late 1950s, British expatriate Jim Wormold is a single father who operates a modest vacuum cleaner business. He agrees to work as a spy to earn extra money to pay for the expensive tastes of Milly, his high maintenance daughter who desperately wants a horse and a membership to the local country club. In order to make his handlers happy and keep the money flowing, he creates an imaginary network of spies. Before long, he is 'spicing up' his reports by claiming to have intelligence on a secret military base in the mountains and even makes detailed sketches of the facility, earning the admiration of London and helping him to attain the coveted status of Britain's top spy. In reality, the images are enlarged drawings of vacuum cleaner parts [23]. The storyline for *Our Man in Havana*, is absurd, but is it any less absurd to think that the American Government could have spent millions of taxpayer dollars investigating the mating calls of crickets and cicadas that were mistaken for a sophisticated attack by a hostile foreign power? Based on the available evidence, we suggest that the answer to this question is an unequivocal 'No,' because as we noted in the onset of this chapter, humans have a remarkable proclivity for self-deception.

The events in Cuba closely parallel historical outbreaks of mass hysteria and social panics, from the clusters of symptoms to the social patterning of victims which was confined to Embassy staff and their families. These antecedents also share another common feature: the absence of concrete evidence. Each of these features point to mass psychogenic illness exacerbated by mundane sounds and ever-present ailments that were framed within the Cold War context of Cuban-American relations. The decision by State Department doctors to consult with a specialist in acoustical weapons was pivotal and was only done because of the presence of sounds and sensations accompanying the symptoms. Descriptions included "a high pitched beam of sound," and a "baffling sensation' akin to driving with windows partially down …" These accounts are ambiguous and more consistent with tinnitus, background noises, and ambiguous health complaints than a sonic attack. We also know that some of the sounds associated with feeling unwell, were insects because they were recorded and identified. The subsequent discussion about a possible sonic attack allowed worried Embassy staff to put ambiguous sounds and symptoms into a new category – a sonic attack, and later when the facts did not fit, a microwave attack. Once this latter possibility was scrutinized, it too lost favor. The creation of 'Havana Syndrome' exemplifies the power of belief. Mass psychogenic illness and the redefining of ever-present ailments are the only plausible explanations that fit the facts. Instead of searching for exotic causes, from the very beginning of this episode State Department officials should have stuck to the mundane. English philosopher David Hume once wrote that 'A wise man, therefore, proportions his belief to the evidence [1].' This was good advice in 1748. It remains so today.

The stigma that continues to surround the diagnosis of mass psychogenic illness must change. For too long, sufferers have been viewed as emotionally disturbed, weak-mined, hypochondriacs, prone to flights of fancy, and worse yet, fabricating symptoms. It is important to acknowledge that the Americans and Canadians who were involved in the Embassy 'attacks,' have been through a frightening and frustrating ordeal. They and their families have had their lives turned upside down. This is also true of the many others who were involved in outbreaks of psychogenic illness found throughout this book, from Hummers to wind turbine sufferers to those with combat syndromes. Our conclusions are not meant to demean their narratives because they are victims and their pain is real, even if the underlying cause is psychological. However, they need to understand that the quickest road to recovery is to change their mental programming by accepting the counter-narrative. This poses a challenge for the victims of 'Havana Syndrome' because of the political nature of the outbreak, misinformation that has been reported by news outlets, on social media, and in scientific journals. However, victims can take solace in the knowledge that the evidence for an attack or exposure to a harmful energy source or pesticides, is virtually non-existent, while the case for psychogenic illness and the redefining of ever-present symptoms, is overwhelming, right down to the political backdrop which germinated the seeds of suspicion. The symptoms that began in Cuba as a result of social paranoia and insect sounds, exemplify the power of belief. That same power holds the key to their recovery.

References

1. Ellis RM. Middle way philosophy: omnibus edition. Raleigh: Lulu; 2015. p. 412.
2. This story illustrates just how fallible human beings are, and the extent to which perception and memory reconstruction is subject to error – two key factors that help to drive mass hysterias and social panics. One of us (Bartholomew) first heard this story in 1981. After writing it down in 2018, he remembered that his brother had tape-recorded the talk. Upon listening to it, he was astonished to realize that the 'dragonflies' had been described as 'insects,' while the elephants were buffalo! In fact, his recall of the entire story was considerably different from what had taken place; the man wasn't even a zoologist but an anthropologist. To read the actual account, see: Turnbull CM. The forest people. New York: Simon and Schuster; 1961.
3. Conner JW. Social and psychological reality of European witchcraft beliefs. Psychiatry. 1975;38:366–80. See p. 367.
4. Stone R. Cuban panel claims stress caused mystery illness. Science. 2017;358(6368):1236–7. (December 8).
5. Golden T, Rotella S. The sound and the fury: inside the mystery of the Havana embassy. ProPublica. 2018. https://www.propublica.org/article/diplomats-in-cuba. Accessed 11 Nov 2019.
6. Hoffer ME, Levin BE, Snapp H, Buskirk J, Balaban C. Acute findings in an acquired neurosensory dysfunction. Laryngoscope Investig Otolaryngol. 2018;4:124–31. See p. 5. Even after these findings were released in December 2018, the State Department continued to post a Level 2 Health Advisory for Americans who were considering traveling to Cuba – an Advisory that erroneously claimed that Embassy employees experienced hearing loss.
7. Dorsey S. Pentagon turns focus to Cuba health 'attacks' amid new findings on American victims. CBS News. 12 Sept 2018. https://www.cbsnews.com/news/pentagon-turns-focus-to-cuba-attacks/. Accessed 22 Oct 2019.
8. Nauert, US Department of State Press Briefing, 28 Sept 2017.
9. Swanson R, Hampton S, Green-McKenzie J, Diaz-Arrastia R, Grady M, Ragini V, et al. Neurological manifestations among US government personnel reporting directional audible and sensory phenomena in Havana, Cuba. JAMA. 2018;319(11):1125–33. https://doi.org/10.1001/jama.2018.1742. See p. 1131.
10. Sample I. Fresh row over mysterious sickness affecting US diplomats in Cuba. The Guardian. 24 Feb 2018.
11. Attacks on U.S. diplomats in Cuba: response and oversight. US Senate Committee on Foreign Relations, Subcommittee on Western Hemisphere, Transnational Crime, Civilian Security, Democracy, Human Rights, and Global Women's Issues. Attacks on US diplomats in Cuba. Video of the complete hearing published 2018 Jan 9. https://www.c-span.org/video/?439474-1/state-department-officials-testify-attacks-us-diplomats-cuba. Accessed 22 Oct 2019.

12. Petrie K, Rief W. Psychobiological mechanisms of placebo and nocebo effects: pathways to improve treatments and improve side effects. Annu Rev Psychol. 2019;70:12.1–12.27. https://doi.org/10.1146/annurev-psych-010418-102907. Although mild traumatic brain injury and post-concussion syndrome often occur together, they are not the same thing. Traumatic brain trauma refers to a specific disease mechanism – brain trauma – whereas the post-concussion syndrome is a grouping of symptoms that often occurs after a head injury. The definition of a syndrome is a set of symptoms that occur together, evolve in a characteristic pattern and respond to the same treatment. Post-concussion symptoms are markedly variable, evolve differently and respond to a variety of treatments.
13. Nelson LD, Tarima S, LaRoche AA, Hammeke TA, Barr WB, Guskiewicz K, et al. Preinjury somatization symptoms contribute to clinical recovery after sport-related concussion. Neurology. 2016;86:1856–63. https://doi.org/10.1212/WNL.0000000000002679.
14. Cantril H. The invasion from Mars: a study in the psychology of panic. Princeton: Princeton University Press; 1947. p. 160.
15. Fradkin EK. The air menace and the answer. New York: The Macmillan Company; 1934. p. 1.
16. Struewing J, Gray GC. Epidemic of respiratory complaints exacerbated by mass psychogenic illness in a military recruit population. Am J Epidemiol. 1990;132:1120–9.
17. Nemery B, Fischler B, Boogaerts M, Lison D, Willems J. The coca-cola incident in Belgium, June 1999. Food Chem Toxicol. 2002;40:1657–67.
18. Chapman S, MacKenzie R. Fainting schoolgirls wipe a $A1bn off market value of Gardasil producer. BMJ. 2007;334:1195.
19. Reist M, Klein R. Why are we experimenting with drugs on girls? The Age (Melbourne, Australia). 25 May 2007.
20. Grimes D. We know it's effective. So why is there opposition to the HPV vaccine? The Guardian. 11 Jan 2016.
21. Faiola A. In Cuba, the great American tourism boom goes bust. The Washington Post. 11 May 2018.
22. There's only one way out for Cuba's dismal economy. The New York Times. 28 Mar 2019.
23. Greene G. Our man in Havana. London: William Heinemann; 1958.

Index

Printed in the United States
By Bookmasters